6/08

your guide to

eczema

your

The ROYAL
SOCIETY of
MEDICINE

your guide to
eczema

Dr Sarah Wakelin
MBBS, FRCP(UK)

Hodder Arnold
A MEMBER OF THE HODDER HEADLINE GROUP

Orders: Please contact Bookpoint Ltd, 130 Milton Park,
Abingdon, Oxon OX14 4SB. Telephone: (44) 01235 827720,
Fax: (44) 01235 400454. Lines are open from 9.00 to 18.00,
Monday to Saturday, with a 24-hour message answering
service. You can also order through our website
www.hoddereducation.com

British Library Cataloguing in Publication Data
A catalogue record for this title is available from the British
Library.

ISBN-10: 0 340 90498 4
ISBN-13: 9 780340 904985

First published   2005
Impression number   10 9 8 7 6 5 4 3 2 1
Year   2008   2007   2006   2005

Typeset by Servis Filmsetting Limited, Longsight, Manchester.
Printed in Great Britain for Hodder Arnold, a division of
Hodder Headline, 338 Euston Road, London NW1 3BH,
by Cox & Wyman Ltd, Reading, Berkshire.

Hodder Headline's policy is to use papers that are natural,
renewable and recyclable products and made from wood
grown in sustainable forests. The logging and manufacturing
processes are expected to conform to the environmental
regulations of the country of origin.

Contents

Acknowledgements   viii
Preface   ix
Introduction   xi

1 **Normal skin and eczema**   1
   What is the skin made of?   3
   What is eczema?   9
   Different types of eczema   11
   What does eczema look and feel
      like?   14
   How is eczema diagnosed?   15

2 **Childhood eczema**   18
   Eczema in newborn and young
      babies   18
   Eczema in babies and children   21
   What is atopic eczema?   21
   Atopic eczema and the home
      environment   30
   Atopic eczema and diet   37
   Adverse food reactions in childhood
      atopic eczema   42

	Infection and atopic eczema	46
	Other types of eczema in children	53
3	**Eczema in adults**	**58**
	Adult atopic eczema	58
	Seborrhoeic eczema	62
	Discoid eczema	65
	Endogenous hand and foot eczema	67
	Venous (stasis) eczema	69
	Asteatotic/wintertime dry eczema	72
	Lichen simplex	72
4	**Contact eczema**	**74**
	Irritant contact eczema	75
	Allergic contact eczema	81
5	**Allergy tests in eczema**	**87**
	Tests for immediate allergy reactions	88
	Tests for delayed allergy reactions	91
6	**Eczema treatment**	**97**
	Topical treatment	97
	Oral and intravenous treatments	112
	Ultraviolet therapy	115
	Complementary alternative medicine	117
7	**Taking control**	**120**
	Coping with eczema	120
	Tips for managing itching	124
8	**Health care for patients with eczema**	**127**
	Types of care	127
	Medical personnel	128
	Prescription charges	131
	The NHS appointment system	131

Further help   132
Glossary   134
Index   139

Acknowledgements

To my loved ones, especially Olivia and Sebastian.

I would also like to pay special thanks to St John's Institute of Dermatology and the Medical Illustration Group UK for giving their kind permission to reproduce the illustrations.

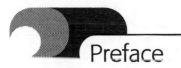# Preface

This new book, published in partnership with the Royal Society of Medicine, provides detailed, useful and up-to-date information on eczema. It contains expert yet user-friendly advice, with such useful features as:

Key Terms: demystifying the jargon
Questions and Answers: answering the burning questions
Myths and Facts: debunking the misconceptions
My Experience: how it feels to live with, or care for someone with, this condition.

Bearing the hallmark of excellence and accessibility that characterizes the work of the Royal Society of Medicine, this important guide will enable you and your family to gain some control over the way your eczema is managed by being better informed.

Peter Richardson,
Director of Publications
Royal Society of Medicine

Introduction

Eczema or dermatitis is one of the most common skin complaints. It affects people of all ages and can start at any time in life. There are several types of eczema, and these have different causes. Although there has been a lot of progress in our understanding of eczema, the reason why most people develop it is still not clear. Eczema is usually very itchy and uncomfortable, as well as being visible to others. When a young child is affected, there can be disruption for the whole family from disturbed sleep and the time taken to apply treatments. In adults, eczema can have a knock-on effect on studies and work, as well as recreational activities and social life.

Eczema is not a trivial problem, and in terms of health-care resources it has been estimated to cost the UK's National Health Service over £125 million a year. Eczema also poses a significant financial burden on affected individuals and their families with the ongoing costs of buying creams and prescription items, as well as lost time at work.

We do not know the total number of people who have eczema, but studies have shown that certain types such as childhood atopic eczema are becoming more common, and it now affects about one in every five children in Europe. For some people, eczema is only a temporary problem, but for many it is a chronic (long-lasting) condition. Unfortunately there is no known cure for most types of eczema, which can make sufferers and their families or carers feel frustrated and fed up. However, this does not mean that nothing can be done – quite the opposite is true. There are now more ways than ever before of helping eczema, and effective treatment is available to relieve symptoms and improve the rash. Ongoing research is leading to new treatments and, as our understanding of eczema grows, it is hoped that one day we will be able to prevent this condition altogether.

The aim of this book is to explain in a straightforward way the different types of eczema, their causes, and the treatment options. This information should give eczema sufferers and their families or carers the knowledge and confidence to manage this condition most effectively. Ultimately, this means that sufferers should be able to cope with their eczema, and learn to live with it rather than letting it rule their lives. There are so many questions relating to eczema, for which our overloaded health-care system does not always allow the necessary time for doctors or nurses to answer. This book will provide the kind of information that people with eczema want and need, without too much medical jargon or scientific detail. I have tried to give clear answers to what are often difficult questions, where a simple 'yes' or 'no' answer is not known. It is written from my viewpoint both as a dermatologist and the mother of young children with eczema. I hope very much that you will find it interesting and useful.

Dr Sarah Wakelin
Consultant Dermatologist
St Mary's Hospital
London

CHAPTER

1

Normal skin and eczema

There is an ever-increasing pressure nowadays to look young and beautiful, and to do so for longer. One of the most noticeable aspects of our appearance is the condition of our skin. Having a healthy skin makes us look and feel good and undoubtedly has a great effect on self-esteem. On the other hand, having a skin complaint can be miserable because unlike other medical problems such as high blood pressure, it is visible for all to see, especially when it affects the hands or face. Few people are fortunate enough to have 'perfect skin' although this is a myth exploded by beauty magazines and cosmetic companies. Most, if not all of us, will get some skin problem or other at some point in our lives, and this can run a long-term or **chronic** course.

chronic disease
A long-lasting health problem, which may be incurable. This term relates to the duration of the disease, not to how severe it is.

More than skin deep – what the skin does

Before going into detail about eczema in its many guises, it may be useful to give you a brief outline of what the skin does. Of course, we take our skin for granted until something goes wrong. If asked to name an important body organ, most people would choose the heart or brain and few would think of the skin. However, without this crucial body part we would literally evaporate and die within minutes. The skin lasts from the earliest weeks of life in the womb until death, and generally does an amazing job. Imagine an item of clothing that would grow as the body grows, last a lifetime and still look good (a few wrinkles and blemishes accepted) after so much washing and hard wearing. Far from being a simple covering, the skin performs many vital functions. One of the most important is protecting the inner body against dangers in the outside world (infections, chemicals, harsh climate and sunshine). For example, the skin makes natural antibacterial substances that prevent bacteria from adhering to it and entering the body. It also helps to keep the internal body temperature constant in extremes of hot and cold, and prevents the loss of internal body fluids and salts. The skin is a large sensory organ, rich in nerve endings that constantly pass messages to the brain about the outside world, and it makes vital body chemicals such as vitamin D while also eliminating toxins. If large areas of skin are lost, for instance, after an extensive burn, the normal functions of the skin are upset and the consequences can be serious. Milder disturbances can occur in people with widespread eczema, so their body temperature regulation is upset, making them feel hot one minute and cold or shivery the next. Skin affected by eczema loses water easily, so sufferers feel thirsty, and their skin is also more vulnerable to infection.

> **Q** I've heard that it's important to drink plenty of water to keep your skin looking good. Can eczema be helped by drinking more water?
>
> **A** As part of a healthy lifestyle, it is recommended that we drink plenty of water and avoid too many dehydrating beverages such as tea, coffee and alcohol. People with widespread eczema need to drink more than usual because they lose more body moisture through their skin. Although drinking plenty of fluids may be of some help in hydrating the skin, what you do to your skin from the outside is much more important — in particular applying moisturizers and emollients regularly (see Chapter 6).

What is the skin made of?

The skin consists of two basic parts (see Figure 1.1):

✧ The outer epidermis

✧ The inner dermis.

The outer layer or epidermis

The **epidermis** is made up of millions of tiny skin cells called **'keratinocytes'** which contain a tough protein called 'keratin'. These cells are constantly growing outwards to the surface, where they flatten, die and flake off. This natural exfoliation usually goes without notice, and it takes about four weeks for a new layer of cells to complete their outward journey to the top layer of the epidermis (see Figure 1.1). If you press a piece of sticky tape against your skin you can remove the

epidermis
The outer layer of the skin which is constantly being renewed and is made up of layer upon layer of skin cells (keratinocytes). These grow outwards to the surface where they die and shed.

keratinocytes
The skin cells that make up most of the epidermis. They contain a tough protein called 'keratin'.

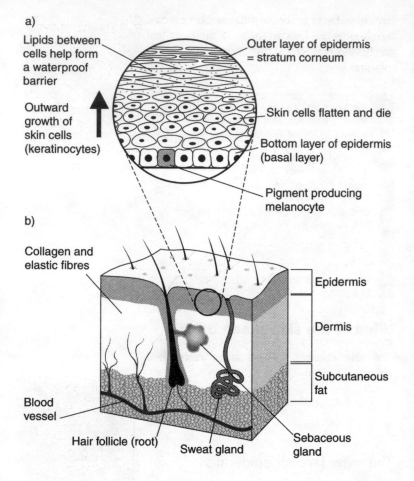

Figure 1.1 a) A magnified diagram of the epidermis (outer layer of the skin);
b) A magnified diagram of the skin.

outermost layers of dead cells, which turn the tape cloudy. This layer of the epidermis is called the 'horny layer' or **'stratum corneum'** and is only as thick as a piece of tissue paper. Nevertheless, it functions as the skin's main barrier, controlling what is allowed in and out. The thickness of the stratum corneum varies considerably from one part of the body to another: it is thinnest on delicate areas such as the skin folds (flexures), neck and face, and thickest on areas prone to friction such as the palms and soles. For example, the stratum corneum is 20 times thinner on the eyelids than on the soles of the feet.

The stratum corneum gets damaged in eczema so the skin quickly loses its natural moisture and becomes cracked and dried out – like a landscape after a drought.

Under the stratum corneum lie layers of skin cells, tightly packed together, and a scattering of pigment cells and some specialized defence cells. The cells of the epidermis are held close together by a special greasy glue consisting of a complex mixture of **lipids**. These include cholesterol, fatty acids and ceramides. If production of these natural lipids is deficient as in some kinds of eczema, or if they are removed by soaps and detergents, the cells shrivel and separate from one another, and they are shed more easily. This reduces the thickness of the barrier layer making the skin prone to dryness, cracking and eczema. These tiny surface cracks allow harmful bacteria to enter the skin, and these can make the eczema worse.

The brown pigment of the skin, melanin, is made by a scattering of special cells in the epidermis called 'melanocytes'. Melanin production increases after exposure to ultraviolet rays in sunshine. Melanocytes transfer this pigment to neighbouring skin cells (keratinocytes) which

stratum corneum
The outermost layer of the epidermis which is made of flat, dead skin cells (keratinocytes). It acts as the skin's main protective barrier, keeping moisture locked in and harmful substances out.

skin lipids
Natural oily substances produced by the skin to help moisturize the outer layer and prevent drying.

grow outwards to the skin surface. This explains why a suntan is temporary, and disappears a few weeks after a sunny holiday. On the plus side, the constant re-growing of the epidermis means that the body can quickly repair damage to this layer as a result of injury or skin disease such as eczema.

The epidermis also contains a network of defence cells called 'Langerhans cells'. These interconnect with one another by long spidery outgrowths to provide an early warning system to detect disease and infection.

The epidermis contains tiny ducts, which carry sweat and grease (sebum) to the skin surface from glands in the deeper **dermis**. Sweat is basically weak salty water, which also contains urea and lactate. These waste chemicals help the outer skin layers retain water, and they are sometimes used as ingredients in moisturizers. They are weak acids and, along with fatty acids in sebum, give the normal skin surface a slightly acidic pH of 5.5.

dermis

The deeper layer of the skin that contains blood and tissue fluid to nourish and heal the skin, and a network of tough and stretchy fibres to give the skin strength.

The deeper skin or dermis

The dermis is the deeper layer of skin under the epidermis and both layers are glued tightly together. The dermis is tough because it contains fibres of collagen and elastin which give the skin its strength and elasticity. Deeply rooted in the dermis are hair follicles, grease (sebaceous) glands and sweat glands. The dermis contains a dense network of nerve fibres and receptors which carry messages of touch, pressure, warmth, cold, pain and itch to the brain. The dermis also contains a rich supply of blood vessels, tissue fluid and lymph vessels that bring nutrients to the skin and take harmful substances away. The amount of blood flowing to the skin varies according to body temperature. To cool the inner body, for example during exercise, skin blood flow increases, allowing heat to escape from the body surface.

Blood in tiny vessels brings oxygen and nutrients to the skin as well as infection-fighting white blood cells. These can pass out of the vessels into the skin and patrol the dermis looking for danger in the form of germs or harmful chemicals. These substances trigger an inflammatory response where more blood and white blood cells get diverted to the skin. The increased blood flow results in redness, heat and swelling, which are the signs of **inflammation**. When the 'battle' is over and the danger has been eliminated, the skin settles back to normal.

> **inflammation**
> A process where more blood cells and infection-fighting substances are present in part of the body. In the skin this causes redness, heat, swelling and soreness or irritation. All these features are present in eczema.

When the deeper dermis is deeply wounded, new collagen bundles are made during the healing process and these cause a scar. Scars are permanent, but usually flatten and fade with time. Although eczema affects the skin's appearance, thankfully it does not cause permanent damage or scarring, unless the skin has been deeply picked or scratched. Repeated rubbing breaks hairs at the surface, and can cause hair loss, but because the hair roots are deeply anchored the hair will re-grow once rubbing stops. Collagen fibres becomes thinner as we get older, which is why elderly people's skin is more fragile, breaking and bruising easily. The amount of collagen is also reduced if steroid tablets are taken long term, or after repeated use of strong topical steroids especially on delicate areas or skin folds (flexures) such as the eyelids (see Chapter 6).

Long-term sun exposure damages the elastic fibres of the dermis so they become a tangled mess. This makes the skin turn slightly yellow and less stretchy, leading to furrows and wrinkles.

Q My son suffered from mild eczema as a toddler. He is now eight years old and his skin is much better, but he has started to get scaly bald patches in the scalp and has a spotty rash on his cheeks. Is this eczema again or another condition?

A Patchy hair loss in children is more likely to be caused by a fungal infection or ringworm than by eczema. Hair loss is unusual in eczema unless the child has widespread involvement of the scalp and repeatedly scratches and rubs. You need to visit your doctor because scalp ringworm needs proper diagnosis and treatment with a course of oral antifungal medicine.

The deepest layer of the skin or subcutis

Under the dermis lies the subcutis which contains a variable thickness of fat – depending on the body site and size. This helps to insulate the body against heat loss, provides a layer of padding against trauma and acts as a fuel reserve in times of food shortage.

myth
The skin is just an outer wrapping for the important internal body organs.

fact
The skin is actually the largest body organ and has an approximate surface area of 2 m² (21.5 ft²) in an adult; it performs many vital functions. The outermost layer acts as a highly effective protective barrier against infection and danger. This layer is dead and constantly being shed so, over a lifetime, the average person loses about 18 kg (39.516) of skin. The skin keeps the inner body temperature constant by sweating and radiating heat. It contains about 5 million sweat glands which can make several litres of sweat every day. There are also about 1 million sensory nerves in the skin, mostly in the face, hands and feet. These constantly relay messages such as touch, temperature and pain to the brain. These vital functions can all be upset in eczema, with increased skin shedding, loss of skin moisture and heat, lowered resistance to infection and over-activity of itch and pain nerves.

What is eczema?

Eczema or **dermatitis** is one of the most common skin complaints. Both words describe the same condition and can be used interchangeably – what one person calls eczema, another may quite acceptably call dermatitis. The word 'eczema' comes from the Greek word meaning 'boiling or bubbling through', while 'dermatitis' means 'inflammation of the skin'.

These names tell us that eczema is an inflammatory skin disease, and that with eczema there are extra red and white blood cells in the skin with a 'cocktail' of natural chemicals called '**antibodies**' and '**cytokines**'. A similar process happens naturally after an injury or burn, and the inflammatory reaction helps to fight infection and heal wounds. However, when this system is activated without an appropriate reason, as in eczema, the end result is an itchy, sore rash. Imagine that the white blood cells are soldiers trained to fight the enemy invaders (bacteria, viruses, etc.) and that they release chemicals called antibodies and cytokines as weapons. If the soldiers start to fight without an enemy they will end up causing unnecessary damage to their surroundings, in this case, the skin. This is a simplified way of thinking about eczema, but it helps to explain why anti-inflammatory treatment such as steroids can help this condition.

The inflammatory process in eczema affects both the epidermis and the underlying dermis. In the epidermis, the keratinocytes (skin cells) become bloated and swollen, making them pull apart from one another. The epidermis becomes like a water-logged sponge, which makes it feel swollen and raised, and the excess fluid can collect into tiny blisters. Chemicals called

eczema/ dermatitis
An inflammatory rash which is red, swollen and blistered, or scaly and itchy.

antibodies
Natural substances produced by white blood cells which help to fight infection.

cytokines
Natural messenger chemicals produced by many different cells in the body, including white blood cells and skin cells. They help to activate defence mechanisms against infection, and aid healing.

'proteases' are activated, and these dissolve the 'glue' that holds the keratinocytes of the outer skin layers together. This makes them shed more easily, causing dryness and increased skin flaking. When the important vital outer layers are lost, the skin is no longer such an effective barrier and tiny surface cracks develop allowing moisture to escape and infections to enter. The increased blood flow in the dermis in eczema causes **signs** of redness (**erythema**) and swelling, and makes the skin feel hot. Inflammatory chemicals in the skin act on nerve endings to cause the uncomfortable, prickly itch (**pruritus**) and urge to scratch that is one of the most distressing **symptoms** of eczema.

erythema
Skin redness due to increased blood flow in the dermis.

pruritus
An unpleasant itchy or prickling sensation that makes you want to scratch.

disease symptoms
The uncomfortable sensations that a person feels, for example pain and itching.

disease signs
The outward appearance of a disease which can be observed by someone else, for example a rash or more specific features such as redness, swelling, blisters, scaling.

myth
People should not touch someone with eczema because it can be contagious.

fact
Eczema is not contagious. Few dermatological diseases nowadays are contagious, although there still appears to be a lot of stigma attached to skin complaints. People with eczema are actually at greater risk of catching certain infections, because their skin is not such an effective barrier against micro-organisms. People who have eczema or other skin problems like psoriasis and acne often feel self-conscious and even ashamed, worrying that they can pass the skin complaint to another person. If someone starts to comment about your or your child's skin, explain politely that the condition is eczema and reassure the person that it is not infectious and cannot be caught.

Q I've never had skin problems before, and have had a terribly itchy rash over all of my body for the last two months. My skin looks dry and red in places and the itch is so bad I can't sleep properly. My boyfriend has also started to feel very itchy and has noticed dry flaky skin between the fingers and small bumps on his wrists and penis. I've tried using moisturizers and some steroid creams but they haven't helped at all. Is this eczema or could it be something else?

A Not all itchy rashes are eczema, and if the problem seems to be spreading to other people you need to see your doctor to check whether you could have a contagious problem such as scabies. This is caused by a tiny parasite that lives in the outer layer of the skin. It is easily cured with use of an anti-scabies cream or lotion. If you do have scabies, it is important that all close contacts and family members are also treated, as they will not have any symptoms in the early stages. If all your close contacts are not treated, you may keep catching scabies from one another and the problem will persist.

Different types of eczema

Although eczema is talked about as if it is one condition, there are several types of eczema. These can look quite different from one another, but all share common features including inflammation. It is important to try and diagnose which type of eczema a person has in order to be able to treat it most effectively and to give an idea of how long lasting the condition is going to be. The different types of eczema are explained overleaf (see Table 1). However, it is not always easy to clarify someone's eczema because it may not fit neatly into of those categories and you can get more than one type of eczema at a time.

Exogenous contact eczema and endogenous or constitutional eczema

There are two main groups of eczema: **Exogenous** or contact eczema and **Endogenous** or constitutional eczema.

exogenous (contact) eczema
Eczema that is caused by skin contact with an external substance.

endogenous (constitutional) eczema
Eczema that occurs due to an inbuilt tendency and not primarily because of something in the outside world.

irritant
A harsh external substance or climate that damages the skin.

allergen
A natural or manmade substance which is misidentified and taken as harmful by some people's immune systems, leading to an allergic reaction.

immune system
The body's defence system which is made up of many specialized cells that circulate through the skin, blood and glands, and has evolved to recognize and fight disease and infection.

Eczema
- **Contact/exogenous**
  Due to skin contact with an external substance
- **Constitutional/endogenous**
  Due to an inbuilt tendency

Different types of eczema tend to affect different age groups so, for example, most childhood eczema is endogenous atopic eczema, while adult eczema is more variable. See Figure 1.2.

Exogenous or contact eczema

This is due to something in the outside world that damages or upsets the skin. The external substance may be natural or artificial. Changes in the climate such as cold dry air can also be included here. If contact with the offending substance is avoided, there is a good chance that the eczema will clear. These external factors can be grouped broadly into **irritants** (harsh things that can damage everyone's skin to some degree) and **allergens** (substances that some people's skin specifically reacts against because their **immune system** has mistakenly identified them as harmful) (see Chapter 4).

The two main types of exogenous/contact eczema are:

✧ Allergic contact eczema

✧ Irritant contact eczema.

Endogenous or constitutional eczema

This is a condition that the affected person has an inbuilt tendency to develop. The eczema sufferer could get this complaint even if they lived in a 'glass bubble' or desert island, away from everything in the outside world. This does not mean that endogenous eczema cannot be made worse or even triggered by things in the environment; but rather that, for reasons largely unknown, the sufferer is inherently susceptible to get this problem. In the same way, some people seem to suffer from headaches or indigestion while others never do. There may be a family tendency suggesting that inherited factors or genes are involved, even though the condition is not visible at birth.

The idea of constitutional or endogenous eczema can be difficult to grasp and accept because people expect skin conditions to have an external reason or identifiable cause. However, most forms of eczema are endogenous in nature.

Table 1 Different types of eczema.

Common types of eczema in different age groups

	Babies/Infants	Children	Adults	Elderly
Irritant contact eczema	+ (nappy rash)		++	
Allergic contact eczema		+	++	++
Atopic eczema	++	++	+	
Seborrhoeic eczema	++		++	+
Discoid eczema		+	++	++
Varicose eczema			+	++
Asteatotic (dry) eczema			+	++

++ Commonest age group
+ Sometimes affected

The different types of endogenous/constitutional eczema include:

✧ Atopic eczema

✧ Seborrhoeic eczema

✧ Discoid eczema

✧ Varicose vein eczema

✧ Asteototic (dry) eczema.

What does eczema look and feel like?

acute eczema
Eczema that has recently started or flared up (over hours or days). The skin is hot, red, swollen, itchy and sore.

chronic eczema
Eczema that has been present for a long time (weeks or months), and is repeatedly scratched. The skin looks thickened, lined and flaky, and feels dry, itchy and sore.

Eczema changes in appearance over time. In the early or '**acute**' stages, hours or days after starting, the skin looks swollen, red and bumpy, and usually feels hot, itchy and sore (see Colour Plate 1). Tiny pinhead-sized water blisters or 'vesicles' may be noticeable and, if scratched, the skin surface breaks easily with weeping, bleeding and crusting. This may clear up within a week or so, after looking dry and crinkled with a flaky surface. If eczema has been present for a longer time, and has been scratched or rubbed, it becomes drier, thickened, lined and darker (see Colour Plate 2). This is called '**chronic**' eczema, and the rather aged, lined appearance is called 'lichenified'. The skin actually thickens, because it is trying to prevent damage from repeated rubbing, just as wearing shoes which are too tight causes corns and callosities.

The edges of eczema areas are usually not clear cut, and it can be difficult to tell where eczema begins, and which areas of skin are normal. This is especially true of atopic eczema (see Chapter 2) where the skin is generally dry all over. Sometimes areas of skin which have been affected by eczema become paler or darker than usual. This is most noticeable in people with dark skins, and will gradually improve once the eczema settles.

Q Our family originates in India. My eight-year-old daughter has pale patches of eczema on her cheeks. I am worried that these are permanent and have been caused by her eczema treatment. What can I do to get the colour back?

A Eczema does not cause scarring or permanent skin damage. People with naturally dark skin often notice that areas affected by eczema become paler or darker than the surrounding skin. Pale patches often occur on the cheeks in children, and dermatologists call this pattern of eczema 'pityriasis alba'. It happens because the pigment cells are taking a rest and making less melanin. The condition settles naturally around the time of puberty when the child's skin becomes greasier. Moisturizers and mild steroid creams may help. Try not to worry about this, as your daughter may pick up your anxieties. The condition should not be confused with vitiligo where the pigment loss tends to be long lasting.

How is eczema diagnosed?

A doctor usually diagnoses eczema or dermatitis by asking the patient all about the rash, and by carefully examining the skin. On rare occasions, it may be helpful to take a small sample of affected skin (a skin biopsy) to be analysed under the microscope, but this is mainly done to rule out other conditions. Usually, listening to the patient (or their parents) and looking at the skin are all that's needed. Diagnosing eczema is relatively simple. It is more of a challenge finding enough time to discuss the causes and triggers of eczema, the different treatments and how to use them effectively, as well as exploring how the sufferer and their family's lives are affected.

Childhood eczema is generally a constitutional or endogenous kind of eczema, and allergy tests

my experience

When I developed an itchy rash on my face, and a scaly scalp, my doctor simply looked at my skin and told me it was eczema and was caused by stress. I had been under a lot of pressure at work but I thought I needed blood tests to look for some internal problem or a vitamin deficiency. The doctor said these were not necessary and prescribed some creams and a shampoo. These helped, although when I stopped using them the rash came back. I asked my doctor to tell me more about my eczema and he explained that I had an endogenous or constitutional type of eczema called seborrhoeic eczema, which can be controlled but not cured with treatment. I was reassured to find that it was nothing to do with my diet and that this sort of complaint is quite common in healthy adults. I've got used to using the treatment now and feel more confident that I can keep my skin complaint under control.

have a limited role and so are not routinely necessary. Face or hand eczema that starts in adulthood may be a form of contact eczema, and skin patch tests may be needed to make sure that a sufferer is not allergic to something such as their cosmetics or toiletries (see Chapter 5). Blood tests are not normally needed for eczema because it is not caused by nutritional deficiencies or internal diseases.

my experience

It's so frustrating looking after a child with eczema. One of the worst things is helplessly watching them scratch and tear at their skin until it bleeds, and the disturbed sleep that this causes for the whole family. One day the eczema settles, and the next it flares up without any obvious reason. I feel responsible and to blame, and the lack of treatment makes me angry and fed up. We hear so much of progress in medicine, even cures for cancer. You'd think that they'd have come up with a cure for something as simple as a skin problem by now."

"You may feel frustrated when faced with a chronic condition like eczema, and this is understandable. The fact that modern science has sent rockets into outer space, but has still not unravelled the causes or a cure for many diseases proves just how complicated the human body is. The skin has an extremely active immune system which is on a constant 'high alert' to detect and protect against infection, and this is over-activated in eczema. Skin diseases are just as complex as heart or lung diseases, and unfortunately a permanent cure is not yet available for most people's of eczema. However, there are plenty of different treatments that make it more manageable, and settle the symptoms. The wide array of creams, oils and ointments may seem confusing at first, but with time, most eczema sufferers or their carers learn how to use these effectively. Only a small minority of children and adults with eczema have a more severe disease that needs hospital-based treatment. Try and keep a positive outlook and find out as much as you can about your or your child's eczema. This will help you to feel more in control of the situation, and more able to cope.

Summary

✧ Eczema is an inflammatory skin disease which looks red, swollen and bumpy, then becomes dry and flaky. It feels hot, sore and itchy.

✧ Eczema can be broadly grouped into external/contact and endogenous/constitutional types.

✧ Repeated scratching makes the skin thickened, and lines and damages the skin surface, worsening the eczema and preventing healing.

✧ Many forms of constitutional eczema are chronic and incurable, but effective treatments are widely available. These need to be continued to keep symptoms under control, just as someone with blood pressure or diabetes takes medication on a long-term basis to stay well. Unfortunately, there is no magic one-off answer for most skin complaints, any more than there is for other medical problems.

CHAPTER

2

Childhood eczema

Eczema is one of the most common skin problems in babies and children, and can cause distress for the child and his or her carers. Thankfully, most cases are mild and can be helped and kept under control by simple treatment which is applied to the skin. Although eczema may be upsetting, it is reassuring to remember that childhood eczema is usually mild and gets better; few children will be affected badly enough to need ongoing hospital treatment.

Eczema in newborn and young babies

Cradle cap

cradle cap
A common minor skin complaint in newborn and young babies caused by a build-up of scaly skin in the scalp.

Shortly after birth, many babies develop **cradle cap**, which is caused by a scaly build-up of dead outer skin. This is usually a mild and temporary problem, and the scales can be gently washed out with baby shampoo after softening with a moisturizer such as aqueous cream or olive oil. Arachis oil is not recommended because it comes from peanuts and may cause peanut allergy. Sometimes a scaly, red rash spreads down on to the forehead and also affects the nappy area. This is called 'infantile seborrhoeic dermatitis'. Although parents often worry, the baby is usually not upset by this skin complaint. Sometimes there may be irritation that causes the baby to rub, and the affected skin may become infected. In this case, a short course of antibiotic cream or medicine may be needed. Cradle cap usually gets better within a few months. Some mild scalp scaling can last for longer into toddlerhood.

Nappy rash

In the days before disposable nappies and liners, nappy rash was an almost universal problem, and it is still extremely common. The rash is caused by the wetness of a nappy rubbing against a baby's delicate skin, which is then irritated by urine and faeces, and prone to infection. Nappy rash is a good example of an irritant contact eczema (dermatitis), i.e. a kind of eczema caused by something harsh in the outside world that comes into contact with the skin. Modern nappies are designed to hold large volumes of moisture and draw fluids away from the skin surface to keep babies' skin dry. Frequent nappy changing (about seven times a day) is the most important measure to avoid nappy rash. Breastfed babies also seem to get less nappy rash than formula-fed babies.

Irritant nappy eczema looks like a minor burn with shiny redness, which settles to leave dry, crinkled, parchment-like skin. It is usually worse at the body sites where skin contact with the nappy

candida

A family of yeast that can infect warm, moist skin areas such as the skin folds around the groin to cause soreness and redness (thrush).

is greatest, that is the curvatures of the bottom and the scrotum or vulval labia (lips). If the rash has a raw looking appearance, extends into the skin folds and has a clear cut-off point with a lot of small red spots close to the edges, this suggests there is infection with a yeast called '**candida**' (thrush). Candidal nappy rash is more common in children who have recently taken antibiotics, and it can also be triggered by diarrhoea.

Other less common rashes in the nappy area include infantile seborrhoeic dermatitis which is usually found in babies who have cradle cap. These babies may also have scaly and red patches under the arms and around the umbilicus. Sweat rash or 'intertrigo' affects the skin folds and is due to trapped moisture, usually in overweight babies. Allergic dermatitis is very uncommon in the nappy area in babies, but can be caused by contact with fragrances, lanolin or antibiotics in lotions and creams. On rare instances, more unusual skin diseases can cause rashes in the nappy area. If things do not get better with the usual treatment (see below), your doctor may recommend that your baby is referred to a dermatologist.

Q My eight-month-old daughter has recently picked up a tummy bug. Although she is not being sick, she has had diarrhoea for two days and has developed a raw-looking rash on her bottom. What can I do to get it better?

A To treat nappy rash, use high absorbency disposable nappies instead of cloth nappies. This will minimize the contact of the baby's skin with wetness. Nappies need to be changed more frequently than usual if the baby has diarrhoea. Do not use any soap or bubble baths because these will upset the skin. Wash the affected area with warm water and a gentle soap substitute,

A then apply a zinc-containing nappy rash cream or silicone barrier cream. Talcum powder should be avoided. It can help to let any raw areas dry out by allowing the baby to spend some time without a nappy, lying on a large clean towel. If there are signs of a candida (thrush) infection, an anti-yeast cream or ointment such as clotrimazole or nystatin may be needed. A mild steroid is sometimes added to these preparations to soothe the inflammation. Products containing steroids should not be applied more than twice a day. If your baby's diarrhoea does not settle, you should consult your general practitioner.

Eczema in babies and children

Atopic eczema

Most eczema that starts in babies over the age of three months and in young children is an inbuilt or endogenous form of eczema called 'atopic eczema'.

What is atopic eczema?

Atopic eczema is the commonest type of eczema and the main type that affects children. It usually starts before school age and typically appears first around the age of between three to six months. Atopic eczema usually affects the cheeks and forehead in babies, then the knees when they crawl, and later the hollows or 'flexures' of the arms, wrists, knees and ankles. Most children also have generally dry skin. Atopic eczema may spread on to the torso and cover a large part of the body, as well as the scalp, and the creases around the ears and eyes. It often spares skin covered by nappies in young children. In adults, the hands and face are frequently affected (see Figure 2.1). Atopic eczema is extremely itchy (see Colour Plate 3).

atopic eczema
An endogenous or constitutional type of eczema that usually starts in babies or children who have a family tendency to eczema, asthma and hay fever. It is extremely itchy and is normally worse in the skin folds.

Infant

Mainly affects face,
patchy on body
and limbs

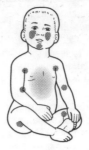

Child

Eczema settles into elbow
and knee folds, around
wrists and ankles, and also
on the eyelids

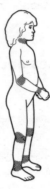

Adult

Hands and face mainly
affected, also wrist and ankle folds
and may be widespread on torso

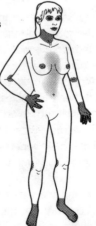

Figure 2.1 Diagrams to show body areas affected by atopic
eczema in different age groups.

Atopic eczema can be confused with other forms of eczema or other rashes, and so research studies now use the following criteria for making a diagnosis:

✧ An itchy skin condition

Plus three or more of:

✧ Rash in the skin creases such as the bends of elbows or behind the knees

✧ Sufferer or their immediate family has asthma or hay fever

✧ Generally dry skin

✧ Rash starts under the age of two years.

What does 'atopic' mean?

The name 'atopic' is used to describe people with a tendency to contract a group of conditions, namely eczema, asthma and hay fever. Individuals with these conditions are also more likely to have food allergies in early infancy. Atopic conditions often run in families, and children may grow out of one problem and into another as they get older. The usual sequence of conditions is food allergy, followed shortly by eczema in infancy, then later on asthma, then hay fever. This has been called the 'atopic or allergic march' (see Figure 2.2). However, most people do not get all of these complaints and only have one or two atopic conditions in their lifetime.

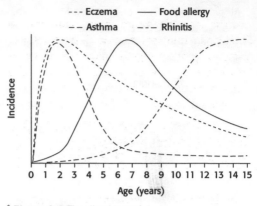

Figure 2.2 The allergic march.

How common is atopic eczema?

It is widely believed that atopic conditions are becoming more common in developed countries, with increasing numbers of people suffering from atopic eczema, asthma and hay fever over recent decades. Recent studies have estimated that about one in every five children in Europe have atopic eczema, while similar studies from the 1940s showed only one in 20 children to be affected. Although this could be partly because people are now more aware that these conditions exist, there does seem to have been a genuine increase in their **prevalence**. The reason for this remains a puzzle, but changes in our living environments are implicated. Most children grow out of atopic eczema so it is less common among adults. Estimates of how many adults have atopic eczema range from two to ten per cent.

Although atopic eczema is increasingly common, it should be remembered that most children only get mild eczema and can be looked after by their doctor without the need for hospital-based treatment. Only a small percentage of children with eczema (1–2 per cent) are severely affected.

prevalence
The proportion of people with a condition in a defined population.

Atopic conditions are more common in developed countries than in less developed countries, and are slightly commoner in towns than in the countryside. Atopic eczema is also more widespread in wealthier families and among children who come from small families.

myth

Children can't have eczema unless one of their parents has this complaint.

fact

Atopic conditions (eczema, asthma and hay fever) usually run in families, but not always. If one parent has an atopic condition then about half of their children will also have an atopic condition. If both parents have an atopic condition, then on average, three out of four of their children will also be affected. Another way of looking at this is if a child has atopic eczema then there is about a 70 per cent chance that a close family member (sibling or parent) will have also suffered from an atopic condition. However, sometimes a child gets atopic eczema without any history of this sort of problem in the family. It therefore appears that inherited or genetic factors are quite important in determining who gets atopic eczema, but they do not provide the whole explanation.

How does atopic eczema affect children?

Atopic eczema can have a big impact on the lives of sufferers and their families. This is being increasingly recognized, and recent studies have looked at the effects of eczema on 'quality of life'. The main areas that affect a child's life are:

✧ Skin irritation and soreness from scratching

✧ Disturbed sleep leading to tiredness

✧ Skin appearance which can lead to teasing or isolation from other children and adults

✧ The need for frequent use of greasy skin applications and visits to the doctor

✧ The need for special clothing and bedding

✧ Avoiding special activities such as swimming and sport.

Children may also have other atopic problems such as rhinitis (runny nose) and asthma. These sorts of problems can also affect older children and adults.

The usual outcomes of childhood atopic eczema can be simplified as follows:

✧ Clears spontaneously and does not reappear

✧ Clears during late childhood/teens then reappears in early adult life

✧ Persists into teens and adult life.

myth
All children grow out of their eczema in time.

fact
Most children who are going to get atopic eczema develop this condition before the age of five, and in half of childhood sufferers it has already appeared by the age of six months. Atopic eczema is mainly a childhood skin condition, and most children grow out of it as they get to their mid-teens. However, it can persist or reappear in adult life. So, even when eczema has apparently cleared, there is no lifetime guarantee that it will not come back again. The fluctuating nature of eczema means that different studies have shown quite widely differing rates of eczema clearance. As a general rule, the more severe the eczema and the earlier it starts, the more likely it is to persist and to be accompanied by other atopic conditions.

Are all atopic conditions caused by allergies?

People with atopic conditions have an increased tendency to make an antibody in their blood called 'imunoglobulin E' or 'IgE'. This antibody evolved over millions of years to protect us against gut infections in early life and parasites such as worms. Why people with atopy make larger amounts of IgE antibodies remains unknown. When they are not fighting parasites, IgE antibodies may be misguided and target other substances in our outside world such as food, drugs, animal fur, pollen and house dust mites. These are called allergens. This misdirected immune action can lead to symptoms of allergy.

Allergies appear to play an important role in some of the atopic conditions, for example, hay fever is clearly triggered by pollen allergens. Sufferers get symptoms of sneezing, watering and itchy noses and eyes within minutes of exposure to high levels of pollen, but do not have symptoms during the months of the year when pollen is not present in their surroundings.

Although atopic eczema sufferers may have allergies to various allergens in their environment, the importance of these in making the skin worse is not always clear cut, and eliminating them does not cure the condition. For instance, an eczema sufferer who is allergic to grass pollen may notice that their skin gets red and itchy shortly after sitting on the grass, or **flares** up the next day. However, avoiding grass does not make the eczema disappear. Similarly, an eczema sufferer who is allergic to cats may notice that the eczema on exposed sites such as the hands and face flares after stroking a cat. Exposure to the cat is therefore an aggravating factor but, once again, avoiding cats does not cure the eczema.

IgE antibodies bind to special cells in the blood, skin, eyelids, nose and airways called 'mast cells'.

imunoglobulin E (IgE)

A type of infection-fighting antibody made by white blood cells which is overproduced in people with atopic conditions. It can trigger allergic reactions when the body comes into contact with an allergen.

eczema flare

When eczema becomes active, looking red and swollen or dry, and feeling hot and itchy.

When these cells come into contact with allergens, a reaction is triggered within minutes and causes the release of a cocktail of chemicals, including a substance called 'histamine'. Histamine causes redness, swelling and itch – just like the rash from a stinging nettle. Antihistamines (see Chapter 6) prevent histamine from working, and are useful in reducing the symptoms of these immediate allergy reactions.

Skin prick tests and blood tests can be done to see if someone has IgE-type antibodies to allergens (see Chapter 6). IgE-type antibodies to common airborne allergens can be demonstrated in 30–40 per cent of the general population, but not all will have symptoms of atopic conditions. People who have extra IgE antibodies are said to be **'sensitized'** to allergens. However, the situation gets a little confusing here because being sensitized does not necessarily mean that the person will have any symptoms of allergic or atopic complaints.

allergic sensitization

When someone's immune system has identified an allergen as 'harmful' and the person is therefore at risk of getting symptoms of an allergic reaction when they are exposed to the allergen.

What causes atopic eczema?

There has been a lot of laboratory research on atopic eczema and this has identified many alterations in the skin. However, the questions of what causes eczema and why it starts as well as why it clears in many children, remain unanswered. It's a bit like someone looking at a cake and identifying some of the ingredients, but not knowing how they were all put together. A similar incomplete understanding applies to many other chronic medical problems. There are two main ways in which atopic eczema skin differs from normal skin (see Figure 2.3):

1 Atopic eczema skin is an imperfect barrier against the outside world. It contains less natural oils and loses moisture more easily than normal skin, leading to surface cracks that

allow penetration of potentially harmful bacteria and allergens. These can trigger an immune response leading to inflammation with itching, soreness and a rash. Scratching damages the skin barrier even further, leading to more inflammation and infection, setting up a vicious circle (see Colour Plate 4).

2 Atopic eczema sufferers have overactive immune systems that are triggered inappropriately by harmless allergens in the outside world such as dust, pollen or animal fur. This again leads to inflammation of the skin with itching, soreness and a rash.

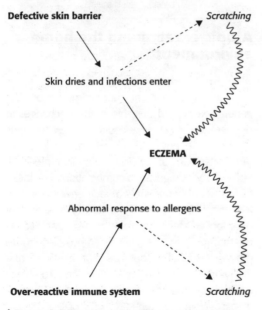

Figure 2.3 The skin abnormalities in atopic eczema.

The various aspects of our environment which may affect atopic eczema will now be considered in more detail.

myth
Eczema sufferers lack oil in their skin and this can be helped by taking supplements such as evening primrose oil.

fact

Although it is true that eczema sufferers usually have a dry skin, the most effective way of treating this is externally with moisturizers, not through dietary measures. The skin of eczema sufferers may lack certain substances called essential fatty acids which are needed to make the outer coat or membrane of epidermal cells (keratiocytes – see Chapter 1). This could be one reason why eczema skin is a less effective barrier and is prone to inflammation. Evening primrose oil and borage oil contain high levels of the essential fatty acid linoleic acid. However, a recent analysis of the results of many studies on these supplements failed to show that they were of benefit in atopic eczema.

Atopic eczema and the home environment

We do not understand why eczema and atopic conditions have become more common, but it is generally accepted that this is due to changes in our ways of living. These could include alterations in our home environment with raised levels of dust mites, lack of exposure to certain infections and dietary changes, or a combination of all these factors. The importance of our environment in triggering eczema is supported by studies that have looked at the rates of eczema in populations migrating from a tropical country to more prosperous cooler countries. For example, one study showed that only one in 20 black Caribbean children living in Jamaica developed atopic eczema compared with one in seven similar children living in London.

The hygiene hypothesis and atopic conditions

Newborn babies have an immature immune system that can be thought of as slightly imbalanced or allergy-prone. Certain kinds of infection in early life may be important in helping the immune system mature, allowing it to focus on protecting us against harmful infections. It has been noticed that the younger children in large families are less likely to have atopic eczema, and children who are brought up on farms have less eczema than those who live in towns. One possible explanation is that these children have more exposure to certain microbes, which helps their immune systems mature properly.

One recent idea which has been put forward to explain the rise in allergic conditions is called the 'hygiene hypothesis'. This proposes that the cleaner homes found in a Western, industrial style of living reduce the chances of 'helpful' infections in early life, so the immune system stays imbalanced and allergy-prone. The immune system then focuses on harmless targets in our environment, i.e. allergens, and this leads to atopic conditions including eczema. Studies are underway to see if giving the right kind of infection in a safe way to young babies can prevent atopic conditions.

Q My husband has asthma, and I have had eczema since childhood. We are planning to start a family soon and would like to do all we can to stop our children getting these problems. Is it possible to prevent eczema and other atopic conditions?

A There is no known way of preventing eczema and other atopic conditions altogether. However, there are several things that you can do to reduce the risk of your child developing these complaints. Exclusive breastfeeding for the first four to six months of life may lessen the chances of getting childhood eczema, and keeping the level of dust mites in your home low can help if the child has already deiveloped eczema. Smoking in pregnancy and exposure to tobacco smoke at home in early childhood, increase the risk of asthma and allergies, so keep babies and children away from smoky places and try to make your home a smoke-free zone.

Q What are probiotics and are they good for eczema?

A Probiotics are health promoting bacteria which are abundant in the gut. It is thought that they benefit the body by fighting off dangerous or pathogenic bacteria. They may also have a calming or anti-allergy effect on the gut. Millions of bacteria start to colonize the gut very shortly after birth. Two important species are lactobacillus and bifidobacterium. People with atopic conditions, including eczema, may have less of these good bacteria in their bodies, hence the interest in adding them to the diet. The natural balance of probiotic bacteria can also be upset by taking broad-spectrum antibiotics. Several studies have looked at whether probiotics could help prevent or treat eczema. One study showed that supplementing mothers with lactobacillus when they are pregnant, and then their infants after birth, reduced the chances of eczema development in early childhood. However, this needs supporting with further evidence. Several studies have investigated the effects of probiotics on young children with established eczema, but these have not shown any convincing benefit. The optimum doses and regimen for probiotics is not known, and they may cause serious infections in debilitated individuals so their use is not yet generally recommended.

Q Should children with eczema have routine immunizations?

A Although a few studies have shown a higher rate of atopic dermatitis in children who had routine immunizations, other studies have failed to show any effect. It is therefore strongly recommended that children with atopic eczema and other atopic conditions should follow a normal immunization programme.

House dust mites

The house dust mite (*dermatophagoides peronyssinus*) is a tiny beetle-like organism that can only be seen under a microscope. House dust mites do not bite and they are harmless except to people who are allergic to them. They feed on fragments of dead skin and are abundant in places where there is a lot of skin debris such as pillows, bed clothes and mattresses. Their bodies contain a high percentage of water which they absorb from the surrounding air. This means that they cannot survive in very dry climates. They grow best in dark, damp, warm environments, and thrive in soft furnishings in well-insulated, centrally heated, carpeted houses. House dust mite levels were lower in the draughty, cold, bare houses that were common years ago. People with atopic conditions have a tendency to become allergic to the faeces (droppings) of house dust mites, and exposure to these can cause allergic reactions.

Dust mite allergy is an important cause of asthma and nasal allergies (rhinitis). Many atopic eczema sufferers are allergic to house dust mites, but it is not clear how much this allergy contributes to their skin condition. Some studies have shown that reducing house dust mite levels in the home can improve eczema, but levels have to be kept extremely low to get this benefit. It is not possible to remove all dust mites permanently, and the 'safe' lower limit for eczema sufferers is unknown. However, house dust mite reduction measures are worth trying, especially for children who have moderately severe eczema. These measures involve the following:

◇ **The bed**. Encase the mattress and pillows with special mite-proof covers which can now be bought at most large department stores. If possible, buy a new mattress and encase it in the covers before use. The covers allow air and moisture to escape but trap mites. Plastic covers are not a good choice as they do not allow moisture to escape and can lead to excessive heat which can worsen eczema. Vacuuming the mattress is not recommended as this simply brings deeply buried dust to the surface. Air the bed before remaking it and, if possible, replace blankets with a synthetic-filled duvet. Use inexpensive synthetic pillows and replace these regularly.

✧ **Flooring**. Choose hard flooring – wood, tiles or lino – rather than carpets. Short-pile carpets are better than longer pile as they allow less mites to be airborne.

✧ **Soft furnishings.** Consider leather or leather-like furniture when you buy new sofas and chairs, as these are easy to clean and wipe. Otherwise, choose items with washable covers. Anti-dust mite (acaricides) chemical sprays can be used, but their effectiveness is uncertain because they leave behind dead mites and their droppings. These sprays should not be used on bedding.

✧ **Indoor temperature**. The ideal temperature for house dust mites is between 17°C and 24°C, so it helps to keep rooms cool and well ventilated. Avoid drying washing indoors as this will increase the humidity. Air the bedroom and living areas regularly.

✧ **Household cleaning**. Remove dust from corners and surfaces regularly using a slightly damp cloth. Vacuum every day with a modern cleaner which has a micro-filter and avoid old-fashioned models with a cloth dust bag. However, it is not necessary to spend a lot of money buying the most sophisticated vacuum cleaner. Do not brush or shake rugs indoors.

⬦ **Laundry**. Bedding should be washed in hot water (at or above 55°) every week. Washing at lower temperatures does not kill mites.

⬦ **Soft toys**. These can harbour dust mites, so choose a cuddly toy which can be hot washed regularly with your child's bedding. Many modern soft toys are only surface cleanable. These can be put in the freezer overnight once a month which will kill dust mites. However, this is not a perfect answer as the dead mites and their droppings persist and can trigger allergies.

Air filters and ionizers are of no benefit in reducing house dust mite levels as the mites and their droppings fall on to surfaces and do not stay airborne for long.

Domestic pets

Atopic eczema sufferers may develop allergies to furry pets, particularly cats and dogs. The allergies are mainly caused by the pet's shed skin or saliva. Once again it is difficult to know how important such allergies are in aggravating someone's eczema.

Houses with cats and dogs contain very high levels of pet allergens, and these remain high for several months after permanent removal of the pet. Sufferers may notice that they get hay fever-like symptoms with itchy eyes and a runny nose shortly after touching the animal, especially if they have touched their faces, and they may also get redness and irritation of the skin. Highly allergic individuals can develop these symptoms just from going into a room where the animal lives. Although most studies have shown that being raised in a family with furry pets increases the rate of atopic conditions, others have suggested that a lot of exposure to pets can have a protective effect, so this is quite a confusing subject. Getting

myth
Eczema is caused by washing powders, and all eczema sufferers should use non-biological detergents.

fact
Although they get blamed for many rashes, it may be a surprise to learn that there is actually no scientific evidence that the enzymes in biological fabric detergents make eczema or any other skin complaint worse. Biological powders are more effective at removing certain stains at low temperature washes, but some people feel that they cause skin irritation. Whatever detergent you choose, be careful not to overload your washing machine, as this prevents the clothes from being rinsed properly, leading to detergent deposits which can irritate delicate areas such as the skin folds. Eczema sufferers should take great care to choose clothing which is soft and absorbent, but they do not really need to worry about how it should be washed.

rid of the family pet can be extremely traumatic, especially for a young child, and this is not routinely recommended. However, the bedrooms and, if possible, the living room should be kept pet-free. Regular vacuuming and choosing hard flooring rather than carpets can help to reduce the airborne levels of pet allergens. Washing the animal thoroughly every week has been recommended, but this is seldom a practical option with cats!

If there is atopic eczema or asthma in the family it may be simplest to avoid getting a furry pet in the first place.

Q I've heard that some allergies can be treated with desensitization. Is this something that can help eczema?

A Desensitization is a way of trying to make the immune system tolerate something that is causing allergy symptoms. It is carried out by repeatedly exposing an allergic individual to increasing amounts of the allergen and is used today for severe or life-threatening allergies such as bee and wasp allergies. Desensitization takes many months and involves repeated injections which cause itchy skin swellings and sometimes trigger severe allergic reactions. Because of this, it should only be carried out under expert medical supervision. It is therefore a slow, time-consuming process. Eczema sufferers may have allergies, but desensitization is not of any proven benefit and does not have a place in the management of this condition at present.

Q Is hard water bad for eczema and should all eczema sufferers install a water softener in their homes?

A There does seem to be a link between water hardness and atopic eczema, although it is not very strong. Studies have confirmed that more

A children who live in hard water areas suffer from eczema. Hard water is thought to prolong or aggravate eczema rather than cause new cases. This could be because you need to use more soap and shampoo to get a lather and this dries the skin, or because the calcium irritates the skin directly. Chlorine in water supplies has also been suggested to cause skin irritation.

Before you consider getting a water softener, first check whether you live in a hard water area. Installing and maintaining a water softening system can be expensive, and any improvement in your eczema is likely to be modest. Whatever the water hardness, eczema sufferers should avoid using soap because it dries the skin (see Chapter 6).

Atopic eczema and diet

Among eczema sufferers and their families there is a tremendous amount of interest in the role of diet in this condition. Many people try modifying their diet in the hope of curing eczema, but unfortunately this is rarely successful. It is likely that in some individuals, certain foods can aggravate eczema and make it worse. This mostly applies to young children under the age of three, especially those with quite severe eczema. Food is rarely of relevance in older children or in adult eczema. Regrettably, a quick and simple test that says 'yes' or 'no' to the question of whether eczema is food aggravated does not exist, and many of the questions regarding eczema and diet remain unanswered. For the majority of eczema sufferers, current medical advice is to follow a healthy, varied and balanced diet, and to focus their attention and energy on using their treatment most effectively.

The pregnant mother's diet and eczema prevention

There have been several studies looking at whether restricting the mother's diet during pregnancy will reduce the chance of her babies developing eczema. These have shown no evidence of benefit, but have shown a possibly harmful effect because the babies were born smaller than usual. It is extremely important that pregnant mothers have a healthy and varied diet in order to provide their growing baby with a good balance of nutrients. Mothers should not smoke during pregnancy because this has many harmful effects on their baby, as well as increasing the risk of allergies. Alcohol intake during pregnancy has also been linked to allergic conditions, and should be kept to a minimum.

Breastfeeding and eczema

The recommendations for allergy prevention are that newborn babies should be fed only breast milk for the first six months. Breast milk is preferable to formula milk because it is germ-free, readily available, and always at the correct temperature. It also contains protective antibodies which give the young baby some immunity against infections. Breastfeeding does not always come naturally, and new mothers may need a lot of practice, help and support in the early weeks after birth to establish a regular feeding routine. Exclusive breastfeeding is physically demanding for the mother as it means not being able to top up with a bottle of formula milk at the end of the day when she's tired and her milk supplies are low. Numerous studies have looked at whether breastfeeding reduces the chance of babies getting eczema and other atopic conditions. Most of these have shown an overall benefit, but there are some inconclusive areas. Breastfeeding probably halves the chance that the baby will get eczema, but does not totally prevent it.

One of the complicating factors is that breast milk is not a simple substance, but contains traces of food that the mother has recently eaten, including, for example, cows' milk. If a baby is at high risk of getting atopic conditions it may be of help if the mother stops eating certain allergy provoking foods such as cows' milk and nuts while she is breastfeeding. A few studies have shown that this reduces the chance and severity of baby eczema between 12 and 18 months. Larger studies are needed to find out whether these results are correct.

Formula milk and eczema

Formula milk is an alternative to breast milk that has been specially modified to contain the correct balance of nutrients for a young human baby. Most currently available formula milks are made from cows' milk and contain cows' milk protein, which can cause allergic reactions. Feeding young babies with cows' milk formula instead of breast milk increases the chance that they will become allergic to cows' milk protein. Because of this, 'hypoallergenic' formulas have been developed in which the proteins are digested or hydrolyzed to make them less allergy provoking. Hypoallergenic formula milks are described as 'partially' or 'extensively' hydrolyzed depending on the degree to which the protein is broken down. More recently, formula milks have been made from the smallest possible protein components which are called 'amino acids'. These milks are called 'elemental feeds' and are the only formula milk that is totally non-allergenic and suitable for babies with severe cows' milk protein allergy.

Unfortunately, extensively hydrolyzed and amino acid-based formula milk is much more expensive than standard formula milk and less palatable because it tastes bitter.

There is some evidence that feeding with an extensively hydrolyzed formula milk rather than with standard formula milk, and avoiding cows' milk-containing foods for the first six months of life may reduce the chance of developing food allergies and eczema in babies who are at a high risk of getting these conditions (i.e. in families where parents and siblings have atopic conditions).

Soya milk is made from soya beans and is therefore a plant product. The protein in soya milk is at least as likely to cause allergies as cows' milk protein, so there are no advantages to weaning a baby on to soya formula milk. It can be used as an alternative in babies over six months old who are allergic to cows' milk and on an exclusion diet. However, there are some recent concerns about the long-term safety of giving soya milk in early infancy because it contains oestrogen-like substances.

Goats' milk is very similar to cows' milk and is therefore not a suitable alternative for babies allergic to cows' milk.

Rice milk can be used as an alternative for older children. It has a good calcium content, but limited nutrients.

Weaning, infant feeding and eczema

The ideal diet for a baby who is at risk of atopic eczema or already suffers with it is not known with certainty, but some experts recommend avoiding cows' milk-containing foods for the first year, with continued breastfeeding if possible, or giving hydrolyzed formula milk. A baby's digestive system needs time to adapt to food, so solids should not be introduced before six months. However, it is important that babies start some solids at this age in order to gain weight and learn how to feed. Babies should be weaned on to puréed fruit and vegetables, then on to an extra energy source such as baby rice or potatoes. Ideally, food should be prepared fresh to avoid artificial colourings and additives, and any convenience foods should be as free from these as possible. Breast or formula milk should still be the main source of protein and fat for at least the first year. It is recommended that infants at a high risk of developing allergies should not eat peanut-containing food until over three years old, but current advice is that all other foods can be introduced gradually after weaning.

Exclusion diets – who needs them?

Babies' and children's bodies are rapidly developing and growing, and therefore it is essential that their diets contain the correct balance of nutrients. For this reason, major adjustments to the diet such as omitting cows' milk – which is an important source of protein and the main source of vitamin D and calcium – should NEVER be undertaken without guidance from a dietician. Well-meaning parents have harmed their children by putting them on exclusion diets without proper advice. A dietician will check that an exclusion diet contains the correct nutrients, and will explain which foods to avoid and how to check ingredient labels properly. Dieticians can give helpful ideas for family meals and snacks as well as advising on how to arrange school meals.

An exclusion diet is carried out for a set length of time, usually four to six weeks. In order to see if it is helping, it is important not to change any other treatment the child receives at this time. The main problem in assessing the effects of an exclusion diet is that eczema naturally fluctuates in severity, and any improvement may have been coincidental rather than because of the diet. If the exclusion diet does not help, the child should resume a normal diet and concentrate on other aspects of eczema treatment.

Exclusion diets are time-consuming and can be difficult to organize in a busy family with other children. Consequently, they are generally only recommended if the child's eczema is moderately severe and not improving with prescribed treatment, or in milder eczema where there is a history that suggests food allergy.

Adverse food reactions in childhood atopic eczema

There are several different ways in which food can upset the body and cause unpleasant reactions. Some of these may be relevant in childhood eczema.

Food intolerance

Food intolerance or hypersensitivity does not involve allergies or the immune system. Examples include, lactose intolerance where sufferers lack a gut enzyme that breaks down milk sugar (lactose) and wheat intolerance, where eating a lot of food, such as bread, causes bloating, colicky tummy pains and diarrhoea. In a similar way, some people find that coffee or cheese gives them a headache. These are adverse or unpleasant reactions but are not caused by an allergy and cannot be diagnosed by allergy tests.

Intolerance to food additives

Many chemicals may be added to food as preservatives or to improve its appearance and/or colour. Most food additives are harmless, for example natural chemicals such as chlorophyll, the green pigment from leaves. However, a small number of food additives has been suggested to aggravate atopic eczema, especially azo colourings and benzoate preservatives. These are now used much less commonly in children's food. Conclusive evidence that food additives are relevant in eczema is lacking, but it may be worth avoiding processed food for a trial period and seeing what happens. Because these are intolerances rather than allergies, they cannot be investigated with allergy tests.

Food allergy

Allergic reactions to food involve the body's immune system and are classified as 'immediate' or 'delayed'.

Immediate food allergy

Immediate reactions occur rapidly, within minutes to an hour or two of food ingestion and are caused by IgE antibodies. Atopic individuals tend to make more IgE and therefore have an increased chance of developing this sort of food allergy. Adults and older children with immediate food allergies often work out which foods cause problems because they get symptoms quickly after eating them, but have no problems if they are avoided. Many different foods can cause immediate allergies, especially nuts, shellfish and fruit. In babies and young children, the most common culprits include milk, eggs, fish, soya, wheat and nuts.

The symptoms of immediate food allergy range from mild itching and swelling of the lips, to more

immediate food allergy
This happens within minutes to an hour or two, and causes swollen lips, hives, scratching, sneezing, wheezing, vomiting or collapse. The diagnosis can be confirmed by allergy tests. Allergy-provoking foods must be strictly avoided.

severe swelling of the tongue and throat, to breathing difficulty. A child may spit the food out or vomit. Other symptoms include a runny nose and sneezing, swelling around the eyes (see Colour Plate 5), wheezing, and a widespread red, itchy nettle rash (urticaria or hives). In severe reactions, sufferers feel light-headed and unwell because their blood pressure is dropping, and they may lose consciousness. This is called 'anaphylactic shock', and it is a life-threatening condition which needs emergency medical treatment.

Although atopic eczema sufferers are more prone to get immediate food allergies, it does not necessarily follow that the food allergy is the *cause* of their eczema. However, studies investigating the association between food allergy and eczema have found that about one-third of babies and young children with moderate or severe eczema also have an immediate food allergy. In these children, avoiding the offending foods sometimes helps the eczema. Immediate food allergies can be confirmed with allergy tests (see Chapter 5) but these tend to overestimate the number of foods that could be troublesome. The management of food allergy is beyond the scope of this book, but it includes strict and careful avoidance of the food, under supervision of a dietician.

delayed food allergy

This happens about 6–24 hours after eating the food, and can cause an eczema flare, scratching, tummy pain and diarrhoea. There is no simple test to confirm this diagnosis, but a food diary may help, and suspect foods can be excluded under the supervision of a dietician.

Delayed food allergy

Some foods can cause slower allergic reactions which appear after 6–24 hours. These delayed food reactions are less clearly understood and more difficult to identify because of their longer time span. Symptoms include colicky tummy pains and diarrhoea, as well as eczema flares. Food-triggered flares may affect some children with eczema, especially these under the age of three. Once again, this does not mean that a food allergy is the cause of their eczema, rather that food is one of several possible aggravating factors.

Similarly it does not mean that by avoiding certain foods the eczema will improve or clear up. There is no simple test for delayed food allergy, and the only investigation is to avoid the suspected food, then reintroduce it and see what happens to the eczema. Keeping a food diary for several weeks can help to identify if there is consistent relationship between a particular food and eczema flares. If there are strong grounds to suspect certain food, an exclusion diet can be tried.

In young children with moderate or severe atopic eczema, it may be helpful to try a diet that excludes certain foods, especially cows' milk protein and eggs for a set period of time (see page 42). It is very important that exclusion diets are only done with the expert advice and supervision of a dietician.

myth
Childhood eczema is caused by food allergy and can be cured by eliminating foods from the diet.

fact
Childhood eczema is not *caused* by food allergy, although young children with eczema are more likely to have food allergies and in a minority these can worsen their eczema.

myth
Eczema is caused by nutritional deficiencies, and sufferers should take vitamin and mineral supplements.

fact
Eczema is not caused by dietary deficiencies. Eczema sufferers, just like anyone else, need a healthy, varied and well-balanced diet, and it is not routinely necessary to take extra vitamins or minerals. If certain foods such as cows' milk protein are being avoided, they may need supplements such as calcium in order to get the recommended daily allowance of vitamins and minerals in their diet. However, in children or adults who have a normal diet, there is no known benefit from taking additional supplements.

Q **My six-year-old son has moderately bad atopic eczema and asthma. He is shorter than most of his classmates, and does not seem to be growing well. He is otherwise a bright and active lad and has a normal diet. Can eczema affect growth, and how can this be treated?**

A Children with moderate to severe eczema often grow more slowly than unaffected children. The reason for this is not clearly understood, but it may

A   be simply because their bodies are using up energy fighting the skin disease. Disturbed sleep can also affect growth. Getting the eczema under better control often triggers a growth spurt during which he should catch up with his classmates. If there is any concern about growth problems in a child with eczema, their height and weight should be carefully monitored (with growth charts) and they should be referred to a paediatrician.

Infection and atopic eczema

One of the most important functions of the skin is to act as a barrier against infection in the outside world. This natural barrier is impaired in atopic eczema making people of all ages who have this skin complaint more vulnerable to certain bacterial and viral skin infections, particularly *Staphylococcus aureus* and *Herpes simplex*. Infections that occur more often in children and adults with atopic eczema are discussed in detail below.

Staphylococcus aureus

Staphylococcus aureus
A bacteria which overgrows on the skin of people with atopic eczema and can lead to eczema flares and skin infections.

Staphylococcus aureus (Staph aureus) is a bacterium. There are about 30 different species of staphylococcus, many of which live harmlessly on the skin's surface. However, *Staph aureus* is a potential pathogen or 'bad guy' which can cause several skin problems including folliculitis (a spotty rash due to infection of the hair follicles), boils and abscesses. Certain rarer strains of *Staph aureus* can cause a crusty yellow rash called 'impetigo', which is highly contagious.

People with atopic eczema are more vulnerable to skin infections with *Staph aureus* because it adheres to their skin more easily, and penetrates through the tiny cracks in the skin surface. This means that virtually all atopic eczema sufferers have *Staph aureus* on their skin. When low levels of bacteria are present and there are no obvious signs of infection, the skin is said to be '**colonized**'. However, *Staph aureus* can thrive and multiply on eczema skin. When the bacterial load increases, signs of infection appear and the eczema flares. See Colour Plates 6 and 7. On **infected eczema** there may be over 10 million bacteria on a patch of skin the size of a fingernail. *Staph aureus* is rarely found on the skin of people who do not have atopic eczema, although they may carry it at certain body sites such as inside the nose without any ill effects.

bacterial colonization
When low levels of bacteria are present on the skin without causing any disease.

infected eczema
Eczema which has an added infection, usually with the bacteria *Staph aureus*. Infected eczema looks red, 'angry' and weepy with yellow crusts or spots, and feels itchy and sore.

Q How can I tell if my eczema is infected?

A Infected eczema looks red, and is weepy with golden-yellow crusts, sore spots and pustules (yellow spots). It may feel sorer than usual, as well as hot and itchy. Because infection-fighting white blood cells multiply in the lymph glands near the infected area, the glands can become tender and swollen. Enlarged lymph glands can sometimes be felt in the groin, under the arms and neck area in people with widespread infected eczema.

Q What is a skin swab and when is it necessary in eczema?

A A skin swab is like a long cotton bud, which is gently rubbed on the skin surface, then analysed in a laboratory. When someone has infected-looking eczema, it can be helpful to take a swab from a weeping area to see what bacteria are present and which antibiotic treatment will work best, i.e. the bacteria's antibiotic sensitivities. This may be particularly important in a person who is allergic to the usual choice of antibiotics. Skin swabs from infected-looking eczema almost always show *Staph aureus*, but sometimes there is an added infection with another bacteria called streptococcus, which should be treated with a course of antibiotics by mouth The swab results usually take several days.

Why is *Staphylococcus aureus* bad for eczema?

When *Staph aureus* proliferates (overgrows) on atopic eczema skin, it boosts the already over-active immune system and can trigger an itchy flare. Scratching causes more damage to the skin surface as well as bleeding and weeping, and this provides an ideal environment for more bacterial growth. This leads to higher levels of *Staph aureus* and a vicious circle of infection and worsening eczema (see Figure 2.4). Certain strains of *Staph aureus* act as if 'turbo charged' and release toxins called 'superantigens', which trigger a very vigorous reaction. The importance of *Staph aureus* in eczema has been shown in experiments where these bacteria were applied to the skin. In normal skin, this application triggered a small patch of eczema, but when *Staph aureus* was applied to the forearm of eczema sufferers, it caused a more widespread flare spreading to the elbow crease.

It is not possible to permanently eradicate *Staph aureus* from the skin of atopic eczema

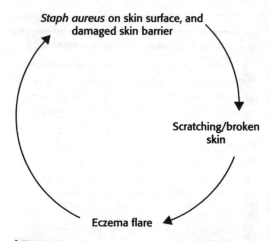

Figure 2.4 The cycle of *Staph aureus* infection in atopic eczema.

sufferers, but levels can be kept low by getting the eczema under good control, and using moisturizers to restore the skin's outer barrier.

Treatment of *Staph aureus* infection

The choice of treatment for *Staph aureus* infection usually depends on how badly the skin is infected.

For milder infections with a minor eczema flare, it may be possible to reduce the level of bacteria simply by treating the eczema actively with moisturizers and topical steroids. Bath oils and soap substitutes with added antiseptics may help reduce infection, and some dermatologists recommend these on a long-term basis in children or adults who have repeated infective flares. Antiseptics that are widely used in eczema products include benzalkonium chloride, triclosan and chlorhexidine. Bathing in a dilute solution of potassium permangonate will dry up weeping infections. Sometimes a topical antibiotic will be prescribed, usually as a combined formulation with a steroid. Several combination creams and ointments exist, but it is best to avoid using them as a long-term treatment because this can encourage resistant bacteria to develop.

If there are signs of heavy bacterial infection with a lot of redness, oozing, crusting and pustules (spots), a course of oral antibiotics is needed. The most commonly prescribed oral antibiotics for treating infected eczema are flucloxacillin and erythromycin. These usually work quickly and the eczema should improve in a few days. However, if other measures are not included to keep it under control and restore the skin barrier, the infection will usually relapse quickly after the antibiotic treatment is completed.

Q I'm 19 years old and have suffered with eczema since early childhood. I've recently had a bad eczema flare on my face with a lot of weeping and crusting skin around my ears. My doctor took a swab and this showed infection with MRSA. She has started me on a course of unusual antibiotic tablets and asked me to come back to the surgery in a week to check that things are getting better. I am quite alarmed as I've read in the papers that this is a serious infection.

A Antibiotic resistance is a very important problem in medicine nowadays, and is one reason why doctors try to avoid unnecessarily prescribing antibiotics. MRSA is the name given to certain strains of *Staph aureus* which are resistant to the antibiotic methicillin (Methicillin Resistant Staph Aureus). The strains are often resistant to other antibiotics and are therefore more difficult to treat because there are fewer options. MRSA infection is not inherently any more dangerous than any other kind of *Staph aureus* in eczema sufferers, but it can cause serious infections in people who are very debilitated or unwell. This mainly occurs in hospitals and, without careful hygiene measures, infections may be easily transferred from one patient to another, leading to an outbreak. This has led to MRSA being referred to as a 'superbug'. Occasionally people with eczema pick up strains of MRSA without any apparent reason. If they are otherwise quite well, there is no special cause for concern, but the correct antibiotic needs to be taken to clear this infection.

General hygiene measures for people with infected eczema at home include the following:

✧ Use antibiotic or antiseptic treatment as prescribed and for the full length of treatment

✧ Bath or shower every day

✧ Use separate hand and bath towels

✧ Avoid face cloths which may harbour bacteria

✧ Change bed linen regularly and wash in a hot wash

✧ Do not prepare food without wearing gloves if the hands are affected.

Herpes simplex and eczema herpeticum

Herpes simplex is the virus that causes cold sores. Most people come into contact with this virus during childhood and have antibodies against it, even if they do not recall ever having a cold sore. Children and adults with atopic eczema are susceptible to a more severe infection with *Herpes simplex*, especially if they have not previously had a cold sore and have no immunity against this virus. It is therefore advisable to avoid direct contact between anyone with eczema and a person who has a cold sore. Rather than getting a single painful sore, eczema sufferers may develop a widespread rash with hundreds of small painful ulcers (see Colour Plate 8). This is called 'eczema herpeticum'. The most commonly affected sites are the head and neck, but it can also spread over the chest and body.

Sufferers usually feel unwell and may have a fever. Unlike a typical eczema flare that feels intensely itchy, sufferers normally complain of soreness and pain. Eczema herpeticum is a potentially serious condition and needs urgent treatment with antiviral medication. It can be difficult to diagnose in someone who has a lot of eczema because the viral sores are more difficult to see. If this diagnosis is suspected, a specialist should be seen urgently. Viral skin swabs can confirm the diagnosis, but treatment with antiviral medication should be started immediately without waiting for the results of these tests.

herpes simplex
This is the virus that causes cold sores. It can lead to a widespread painful infection in children or adults with atopic eczema called 'eczema herpeticum'.

My seven-year-old daughter Lucy has had eczema since she was a baby. Although it was quite bad when she was a toddler, her eczema has got better over the past few years and we can usually keep her comfortable with plenty of moisturizers and occasionally using a steroid ointment. One morning Lucy complained that her skin felt hot and sore, and we noticed that she had a nasty rash on her cheeks and neck, which looked like bad eczema with lots of small spots. She felt unwell and didn't want to get out of bed or eat breakfast. We checked her temperature and found she had a fever of 38 °C. We gave her paracetamol and called the doctor who visited later that morning. He was concerned about Lucy and arranged for her to be seen in the casualty department of our local hospital. She was examined by several doctors, including a paediatrician and a dermatology registrar, and was admitted to the children's ward. We were alarmed that Lucy needed to go into hospital, but the doctors explained they thought she had a severe infection with the cold sore virus. They told us that this can sometimes happen to eczema sufferers, even if their eczema is mild, and it is called 'eczema herpeticum'. Lucy was given an antiviral drug called 'aciclovir' through a drip in her arm for two days, and then a course of tablets. She had some blood tests and a skin swab, which confirmed that she had an infection with the cold sore virus, *Herpes simplex*. Lucy was allowed home after a week when she was feeling much better and her sores were starting to heal. It took several more weeks for the rash to clear up and after this her skin was thankfully back to normal.

Viral warts and Molluscum contagiosum

Warts and Molluscum contagiosum are common childhood infections. Both are caused by viruses, which are tiny germs that are too small to see with an ordinary microscope. Warts are extremely common and mainly affect the hands and feet (verrucas). They sometimes spread to the face, especially around the nose and lips. The wart virus makes the epidermis overgrow, causing the raised, thickened bumps on the skin surface that we recognize as warts. These may have tiny finger-like projections and black dots. Molluscum contagiosum are usually more widespread than warts and appear as small, smooth, red or flesh-coloured bumps, each with a tiny dimple in the centre. They often develop on eczema-prone areas such as the skin folds behind the knees. Many children get warts or Molluscum contagiosum, but these may be slightly more common in atopic eczema sufferers.

Unlike bacterial infections which can be cleared with antibiotics, there are no specific medicines which kill these viruses. It is ultimately up to the body's own immune system to get rid of these infections, and this can take many months. Treatments such as freezing with liquid nitrogen (cryotherapy), may encourage the immune system to fight the infection, but they do not guarantee a cure, and can be painful. Young children do not usually tolerate freezing treatment, unless a local anaesthetic cream is applied to the skin beforehand. Wart paints are a useful alternative for the hands and feet, but it may be simplest to just wait for the infection to clear naturally.

Molluscum contagiosum often become red and crusted when the body's immune system is starting to fight against them. This can look alarming especially if surrounded by eczema, however, it is generally a good sign and means that they are going to clear up soon.

Other types of eczema in children

As mentioned earlier, atopic eczema is by far the commonest form of eczema in children. However, there are other types of eczema which can occur alone or in combination with atopic eczema.

Allergic contact eczema

Allergic contact eczema is one of the external or exogenous types of eczema, i.e. caused by skin contact with a substance in the outside world. It can affect people of all ages, and start at any time in life. It is caused by an over-reaction of the skin's immune system to an otherwise harmless substance or 'allergen' and is discussed in more detail in Chapter 4. The skin has to be exposed to the allergen on more than one occasion, and usually many times, before an allergy develops. Allergic contact dermatitis is extremely rare in babies and uncommon in children under the age of two because they have not come into contact with the allergen enough times.

Similar allergens cause allergic contact eczema in children and in adults. They include nickel in metal jewellery, fragrances and preservatives in toiletries, the ingredients of medicated creams and moisturizers, and substances found in footwear such as leather, rubber and glues. Sometimes it is easy to suspect that someone has allergic contact eczema. For example, allergic contact eczema from the metal nickel in pierced earrings or a belt buckle will only affect areas of skin in contact with these items, and the rash gets better when they are not worn. However, the diagnosis can be overlooked easily in a child who has underlying atopic eczema.

What does allergic contact eczema look like?

Allergic contact eczema looks like other types of eczema, with redness and small blisters in the early phase followed by dryness and flaking skin. Like atopic eczema, it is usually very itchy. Although the rash itself looks like other types of eczema, allergic contact eczema tends to be more patchily distributed on the body, for example shoe allergy only affects the feet. One of the most important steps in diagnosing allergic contact dermatitis in childhood, as in any other age, is to consider it in the first place! The diagnosis of childhood allergic contact eczema should be considered in the following situations:

✧ Their eczema is localized or especially worse on the hands and/or feet

✧ Eczema appears on areas other than the elbow, wrist, knee or ankle creases

✧ If underlying eczema (endogenous) worsens within a few days of using prescribed topical treatment (cream/ointment/eye-drops), moisturizers, sunscreens or toiletries

✧ Eczema occurs at the site of contact with metal items such as earrings, bangles and belt buckles.

Q **My five-year-old daughter has had quite bad eczema since she was a toddler, and has been diagnosed as having atopic eczema. I've heard that children with eczema should have patch tests to find out their allergies. Is this true and how can I get these done?**

A Patch tests are not routinely necessary or helpful in children with an inbuilt or constitutional type of eczema such as atopic eczema; they will not help to uncover the cause of this condition. Patch tests can only diagnose or exclude allergic contact eczema. It is difficult to carry out patch tests in children or adults who have widespread eczema because the patches do not stick well against the skin, and the patches often aggravate the eczema because the skin is covered up for several days. In addition, the patches need to be applied to normal looking skin, otherwise it is very hard to tell which is the person's own underlying eczema and which is an allergic reaction. All this said, if there is a reason to suspect that your daughter could have an additional allergic contact eczema as well as atopic eczema, then patch testing should be considered, and she should be referred to a dermatologist.

The diagnosis of allergic contact eczema is made by patch testing (see Chapter 5). Patch tests can be carried out on children from the age of two years. It is very seldom necessary to patch test babies for the reasons mentioned earlier. Patch testing is not painful but the patches feel sticky and restrictive. It can help young children feel more relaxed if a favourite teddy or doll also has some patches applied at the same time.

Lip lick eczema

Lip lick eczema sometimes causes problems in children and results from the habit of repeatedly licking the lips and surrounding skin. The affected areas become dry and sore, and the rash only extends as far as the tongue can reach. It is usually worse in cold, dry weather and may improve naturally in the summer. The key to treating this problem is to break the habit of lip licking. Although licking sore lips provides instant comfort, it is a bad thing to do because it leads to further dryness. An emollient and mild topical steroid ointment can also be useful. Repeated use of flavoured lip balms can make things worse as the pleasant taste encourages lip licking.

Juvenile plantar dermatitis/eczema

This is an unusual form of eczema that affects the soles or 'plantar' aspect of the feet. It mainly affects children between the ages of 7 and 14, and is thought to be caused by prolonged wearing of trainers with synthetic linings and synthetic socks. The skin becomes sore, red and cracked and has a very characteristic shiny appearance. It seems to get better spontaneously around puberty. Changing to lighter, 'breathable' footwear should help, and mild steroid creams and emollients can be used to relieve any irritation.

CHAPTER

3

Eczema in adults

In adults, eczema is more variable than in children, with a wider range of patterns and causes (as discussed in Chapter 2). Types of adult eczema include both endogenous (constitutional/inbuilt) and exogenous (external/contact) eczema. It is not unusual to have mixed types of eczema, and some adult eczema does not fit neatly into any particular category. The way in which doctors classify eczema is based upon observation of different disease patterns, but skin diseases have been around for much longer than medical textbooks, and do not always follow the 'rules'.

Adult atopic eczema

Atopic eczema is discussed in detail in Chapter 2, and it is an endogenous from of eczema. Most adults with atopic eczema will have had this problem in childhood, but it can occasionally appear for the first time in later life. There may be a history of asthma and hay fever, but these are not essential for making the diagnosis. The main areas of the body that are affected are the hands, neck and face, especially the eyelids. There may be widespread milder eczema and dryness on the torso, and eczema around the wrists, elbows, knees and ankles as in childhood. The nipples are also commonly affected in women.

Atopic eczema is extremely itchy, and this can have a great impact on the sufferer's life. Sleep can be disturbed, leading to daytime fatigue, and flare-ups are particularly awkward because they can occur with little warning and may mean taking time off work or disrupting studies.

Atopic eczema usually fluctuates in severity. Sometimes it is possible to identify an external trigger such as a change in the climate or a stressful event which has caused a flare-up, but often there is no obvious reason. The following are common triggers for adult eczema flares:

◇ Exposure to skin irritants, especially on the hands

◇ Low humidity/air conditioning

◇ Extremes of temperature

◇ Sweating

◇ Skin infections, especially *Staph aureus* (see Chapter 2, page 46)

◇ Emotional or psychological stress and fatigue

◇ Exposure to airborne allergens (house dust mites, animal fur, pollen).

The hands and face are particular trouble zones for adult atopic eczema. This is probably because they are constantly exposed to the outside world and get more than their fair share of contact with allergens and irritant substances.

myth
Adults with eczema often have food allergies which aggravate or cause their eczema.

fact
Dietary allergies and intolerances do not play an important role in causing or aggravating adult eczema. Food allergies can be of some relevance in babies and young children with atopic eczema, but most of these allergies disappear later in childhood. Although some adults are genuinely allergic to food, there does not seem to be any consistent link between this problem and any sort of adult eczema.

Atopic hand eczema

Because adults do so much with their hands, eczema at this site is very troublesome, and it is often a chronic (persistent) problem. The skin in atopic eczema is vulnerable to the drying and damaging effects of irritant substances. This can cause particular difficulties in occupations that involve manual work and exposure to irritants such as catering, cleaning and construction. Certain types of work are best avoided by people who have atopic eczema, especially if they have had problems with their hands in childhood. This needs to be considered when older children and adolescents are planning their careers. Occupations at risk of skin irritation are discussed in more detail in Chapter 4. Even when their hand eczema has cleared, people with atopic eczema have more lines and creases, making the skin look 'old'. This is due to eczema-related dryness of the skin and not because of steroid treatment, as is sometimes suspected.

Another problem with the imperfect skin barrier of atopic eczema is that it allows allergens to penetrate more easily. Certain immediate type allergens can cause particular problems in atopic hand eczema sufferers. These include latex proteins in rubber latex gloves and food protein in meat, fish, fruit and vegetables. Exposure to these allergens can cause immediate reactions with itchy red bumps within minutes, followed later by a worsening of the eczema. The more contact an atopic eczema sufferer has with these sorts of allergens, the more likely it is that they will become allergic to them (more details about immediate type allergens and allergy tests are found in Chapter 5).

my experience

I had quite bad eczema as a child and I remember having problems with my hands, especially doing arts and crafts at school. Thankfully my eczema cleared up in my teens, although it's never really gone from my hands. Until recently I'd been able to keep this under control with moisturizers. However, things got much worse about six months after I took a job as a hotel cleaner. My hands became very sore and dry, and I was finding it difficult to carry on at work. Everything I did with my hands felt awkward and uncomfortable. There were tiny water blisters along the sides of my fingers which were unbearably itchy. I noticed that the rubber gloves I'd been wearing made my hands feel hot and uncomfortable, and I'd get red bumps on the back of my hands about ten minutes after putting them on.

My doctor prescribed a strong steroid ointment and an emollient for hand washing instead of the antibacterial liquid soap I'd been using. She advised me to wear hypoallergenic PVC gloves and, after a few weeks, my skin started to calm down, but I needed to keep using the topical steroids most days to keep it under control. I was referred to a dermatologist, and she diagnosed that, on top of my life-long eczema, I had developed an irritant dermatitis from detergents and cleaning chemicals at work. She also suspected that I had a latex allergy, so I had some patch tests and skin prick tests. The prick tests confirmed that I was allergic to latex in my rubber gloves, and this explained why my hands felt so uncomfortable when I wore them. I'd noticed for some time that my lips and throat felt itchy when I ate Kiwi fruit, and the doctor explained that tropical fruits like Kiwi, banana and avocado have similar proteins to latex, so these allergies often occur together. She advised me to avoid direct skin contact with natural rubber latex items, especially gloves, condoms and balloons. My doctor has been informed about my latex allergy and I told my dentist so he can wear non-latex gloves when I have a check-up. I've now gone back to full-time education and my hands are much better, although they still get dry and cracked very easily, and I need to use a steroid cream from time to time.

Atopic facial eczema

The facial area, in particular the eyelids, is a common trouble zone for adults with atopic eczema. Because the eyelid skin is thinner than the rest of the body, allergens such as dust mites or pollens can penetrate this area more readily and trigger flares. Adults with atopic eczema that mainly affects exposed skin areas may be more likely to have allergies to airborne allergens such as house dust mites, and may benefit from taking steps to reduce contact with these allergens (see Chapter 2, page 33).

Other substances that come into contact with the eyelids such as cosmetics and toiletries can irritate the skin even more and should be avoided. Mascara and liquid foundation or eye liners can be particularly irritating, while eye pencils tend to cause fewer problems. Topical steroids should be used with care around the eyes because the skin here is vulnerable to thinning.

Seborrhoeic eczema

Seborrhoeic eczema is another common type of constitutional eczema that affects the greasy zones of the body. The term 'seborrhoea' literally means 'flowing with **sebum**' (skin grease). This condition occurs briefly in infancy when the baby's grease glands are temporarily activated by its mother's hormones. Seborrhoeic eczema does not affect children, but it can start after puberty when the skin's grease glands become active. The most commonly affected areas are the scalp, eyebrows, the edges of the eyelids, inner cheeks and sides of the nose – areas next to the oily 'T-zone' of the face (see Colour Plate 9). The skin folds around the ears and ear canals can be affected. The upper back

sebum

Skin grease which is made by sebaceous glands in the skin. These glands become active at puberty and are abundant on the face, scalp and upper torso.

and chest are also common sites as well as the larger skin folds around the axillae (armpits), under the breast, and the skin around the genitals.

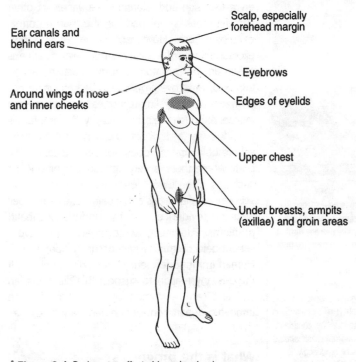

Scalp, especially forehead margin

Ear canals and behind ears

Eyebrows

Around wings of nose and inner cheeks

Edges of eyelids

Upper chest

Under breasts, armpits (axillae) and groin areas

Figure 3.1 Body areas affected by seborrhoeic eczema.

Affected areas appear pink-red and dry, with fine peeling or flaking on the surface. Seborrhoeic eczema is not always itchy, except on the scalp or when the rash is widespread. Dandruff is actually mild seborrhoeic eczema. It appears as tiny white skin flakes with a dry looking scalp. In more severe cases, there may be thicker scaling and redness which can resemble another scaly skin complaint called '**psoriasis**'.

psoriasis
A skin complaint that causes red patches with thick silvery scales and cracks. It usually affects the skin over joints and the scalp, and often runs in families.

pityrosporum

A yeast which normally lives on oily areas of skin. If the natural balance of microbes on the skin is upset, the yeast can overgrow and trigger seborrhoeic eczema.

myth

Seborrhoeic eczema is caused by food and drink, such as bread and beer, which have a high content of yeast.

fact

There is no evidence that dietary yeast is of any importance in any form of eczema. An overgrowth of the skin yeast pityrosporum is thought to trigger seborrhoeic eczema in susceptible people, which is why anti-yeast medication is used to treat this complaint. Pityrosporum yeasts should not be confused with candida which are a different type of yeast that thrive on moist mucosal skin areas and cause thrush.

What causes seborrhoeic eczema?

The cause of seborrhoeic eczema is unknown, but it appears to be due to an overgrowth of a yeast called **'pityrosporum'**. This particular yeast thrives on greasy skin and, along with a variety of other bacteria, makes up part of the skin's normal microbial flora. However, if the yeast grows excessively and this delicate microbial balance is upset, an inflammatory eczema reaction can be triggered. Yeast overgrowth may be encouraged by changes in the climate, sweating, stress and fatigue. Although the skin looks dry, the problem is not due to a lack of oil. On the contrary, seborrhoeic eczema does not affect areas of the body where there is very little sebum production such as the lower legs. People who have seborrhoeic dermatitis are usually quite fit and well with no evidence of any underlying health problems. However, widespread and severe seborrhoeic dermatitis can occur in people with Human Immunodeficiency Virus (HIV) infection. If there is any reason to suspect this diagnosis, an HIV test can be carried out in full confidence through a department of genito-urinary medicine.

What is the prognosis?

Seborrhoeic dermatitis usually runs a chronic course over many years. It may clear completely for periods of time or persist in a mild form with occasional flares. Seborrhoeic dermatitis can start at any point in adult life but is most common between the ages of 18 and 40, and affects more men than women. It may appear for the first time in the elderly. There is no cure, but regular treatment can keep this condition under control.

What sorts of treatment are available?

Because the overgrowth of pityrosporum yeast is thought to be a key factor in seborrhoeic dermatitis, most work by treatments reducing the levels of this yeast. The scalp can act as a reservoir of yeast, so regular use of an anti-yeast shampoo is recommended. Several suitable 'anti-dandruff' shampoos can be bought without prescription. They can also be useful as body washes on hairy backs and chests, but should not be left on the skin as they will cause irritation. Anti-yeast creams can also be used and these are sometimes combined with a mild topical steroid. These dual-action preparations reduce the yeast levels and help to settle the inflammatory process at the same time.

Discoid eczema

Discoid eczema is one of the less common types of endogenous eczema. It mainly affects the arms and legs, and sometimes the hands. This kind of eczema appears as round (discoid) coin-sized, red, scaly patches (see Colour Plate 10). It is most common in middle-aged men. Discoid eczema is very itchy and a relatively strong topical steroid is usually needed to settle the symptoms. As with treatment of other types of endogenous eczema, this is not a cure. Discoid eczema can last for many months, and in some cases comes and goes over several years. Sometimes there is an added bacterial infection and the affected areas get redder, crusted and weepy. In this situation, a combination strong steroid–antibiotic cream can be helpful. The cause remains a mystery, but there is no known link with other health problems or food allergy, and blood tests are unnecessary. It may be confused with other skin complaints that cause red scaly patches such as psoriasis or ringworm (**tinea** fungal infection).

tinea
A ringworm-type fungus that can infect the outer layers of the skin, nails and hair.

Q I've recently developed an itchy circular scaly rash on my feet and shins. A friend suggested it was ringworm, so I tried using an antifungal cream that we had in our medicine box. Although this seemed to relieve some of the dryness it didn't really help, so I bought some mild steroid cream from the chemist. This hasn't worked either, and the rash is now spreading on to my arms. What could it be?

A The commonest causes of itchy, scaly, ring-shaped rashes are eczema and tinea, which is the medical term for a ringworm fungal skin infection. It can be difficult to tell these conditions apart, but if the skin is examined thoroughly your doctor may find helpful clues. People with tinea on the body very often find this fungus on their feet in the form of 'athlete's foot'. This usually causes peeling, cracked white skin between the toes, and flaking skin around the edges of the feet. The toenails may also be infected with tinea, which turns them thick and yellowish-white. Another favourite place for tinea fungal infections in adults is the groin creases. Skin which is infected with tinea is usually itchy and uncomfortable, with a redness and flaking, and these symptoms and signs can mimic eczema.

In order to confirm a diagnosis of tinea, skin samples can be sent for fungal testing (**mycology**). This is done by painlessly scraping a blunt blade across the skin surface to remove the dry outer layers of skin where this fungus lives. The skin samples are inspected under a microscope to see if there is any visible fungus, then cultured in an incubator for several weeks. The same process can be carried out on nail clippings if a tinea nail infection is suspected. The culture results take up to a month, so it can be helpful to use a combination steroid—antifungal treatment which would treat both eczema and tinea in the meanwhile.

If the mycology tests are negative and there are no signs of tinea elsewhere on the body, it is very unlikely that the rash is caused by a fungal infection. In this case it is probably discoid eczema or another red scaly skin complaint such as psoriasis.

mycology tests
Analysis for fungal infections, usually done on scrapings of the skin or nail clippings.

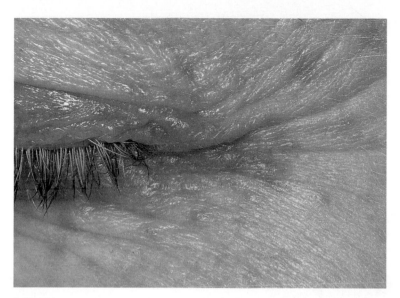

Colour Plate 1
Acute eczema on the outer eyelids.

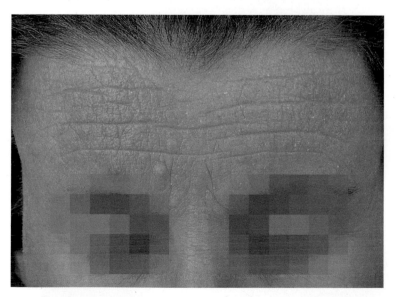

Colour Plate 2
Chronic eczema - showing thickened lined skin (lichenification).

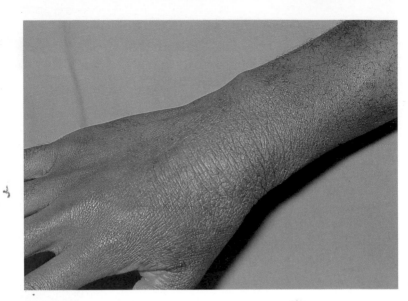

Colour Plate 3
Chronic atopic eczema affecting the wrist.

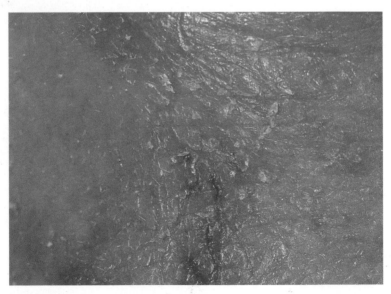

Colour Plate 4
Close-up of inflamed skin in atopic eczema, showing dryness, flaking and surface cracks.

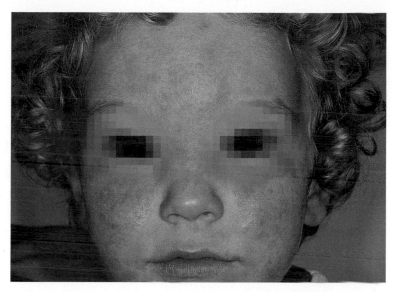

Colour Plate 5
Urticaria caused by an immediate allergy to fish in a child with eczema.

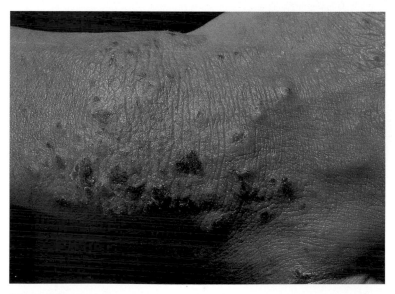

Colour Plate 6
Infected eczema.

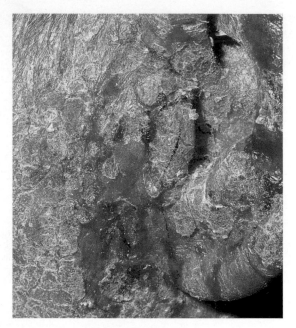

Colour Plate 7
Severely infected eczema around the ear.

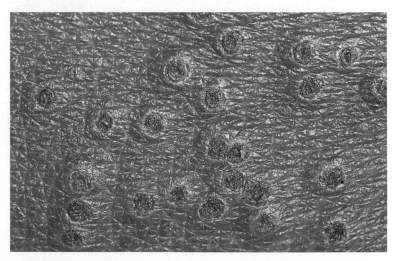

Colour Plate 8
Close-up of eczema herpeticum showing many small uclers (cold sores).

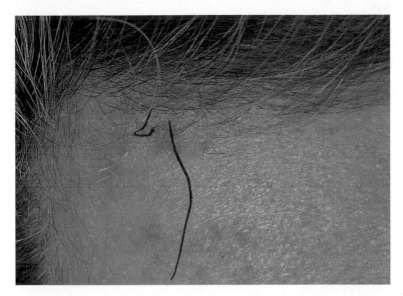

Colour Plate 9
Seborrhoeic eczema affecting the scalp and forehead.

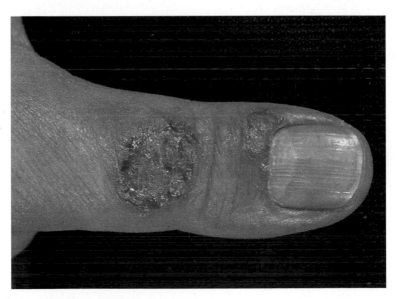

Colour Plate 10
Discoid eczema.

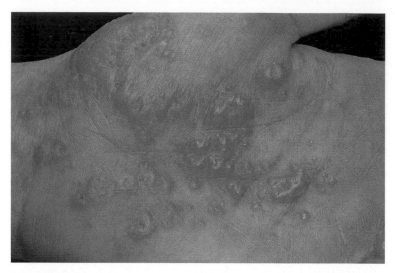

Colour Plate 11
Pompholyx (blistering) hand eczema.

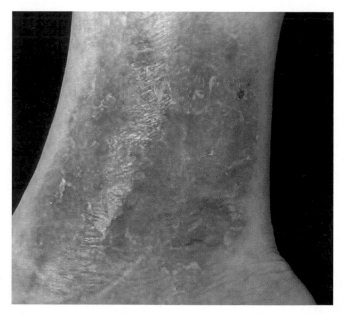

Colour Plate 12
Venous (stasis) eczema around the inner ankle.

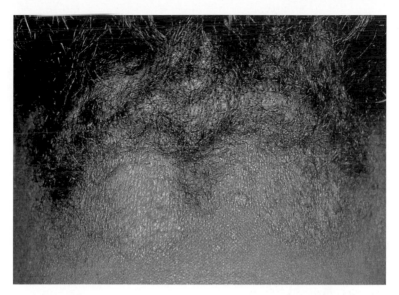

Colour Plate 13
Lichen simplex on the back of the neck.

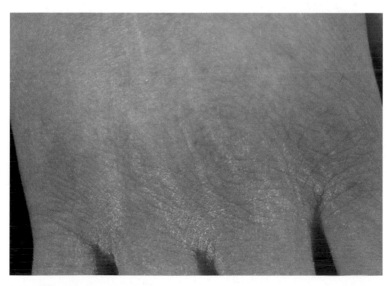

Colour Plate 14
Irritant hand eczema showing dryness and chapping on the back of the hands, especially between the fingers.

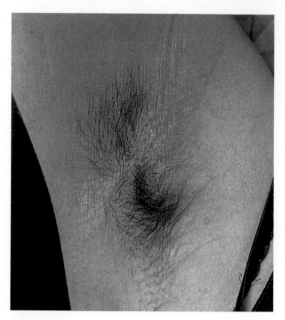

Colour Plate 15
Allergic contact eczema from fragrance in a deodorant.

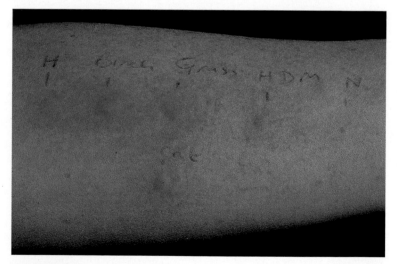

Colour Plate 16
Prick testing with airborne allergens to investigate immediate allergies.

Endogenous hand and foot eczema

Adult hand eczema is the most complicated type of eczema to diagnose because there are several different types and these often co-exist. It is more debilitating than eczema on other body areas because we do so much with our hands. When assessing someone with hand eczema, the doctor needs to know what they do with their hands every day – at work, at home and in relation to hobbies – in order to decide if there are external or contact factors that could be important. For example, someone who develops hand eczema after retiring and notices that their hands get worse the day after doing a lot of gardening could have developed an allergy to plants. It can be very difficult to say whether a contact allergy is causing hand eczema, and so patch tests (see Chapter 5) should be considered for anyone who has a severe or persistent complaint.

The skin on the soles of the feet is very similar to the palms, so eczema that affects one of these sites often affects the other. Several different patterns of endogenous (constitutional) hand and foot eczema are recognized, as detailed below.

Pompholyx (blistering) hand and foot eczema

This is an intensely itchy form of eczema with lots of fluid-filled blisters. These usually appear on the sides of the fingers or feet, and tend to be worse in hot weather. The cause is not known, but it may be related to increased sweating. The blisters are usually small at first, like tiny beads, but they can join together and sometimes reach the size of a fingernail (see Colour Plate 11).

When there are many weepy blisters, it may be helpful to dry the skin by soaking in a mild antiseptic such as a dilute solution (1 in 10,000) of potassium permangonate. Strong steroid creams are usually needed to settle the inflammation and itch, or in severe cases, a short course of steroid tablets.

Hyperkeratotic (thick skin) hand and foot eczema

This type of eczema causes thick, hard areas of skin on the palms and soles of the feet. The centre of the palms and heels are commonly affected, and the thickened skin often has deep surface cracks or fissures. These are very uncomfortable when the skin moves, causing pain on walking and when doing tasks with the hands. It can be helpful to apply a hypoallergenic tape to close the cracks, and a special tape that contains a strong steroid can be obtained on prescription. Moisturizers with added ingredients, such as lactate and urea, can help to soften the brittle hard skin and reduce cracking. Weak, topical steroids are usually ineffective on the thick skin of the palms and soles, so stronger steroids are often prescribed. These can work better if applied for a few weeks under an **occlusive dressing**. 'Occlusion' or covering the skin makes it moist and soft, which allows treatment to get through more easily (just think how soggy and soft the skin on your finger gets if it is covered with a sticking plaster for a day). Cling film can be used as a home-made occlusive dressing, and kept in place over night with surgical tape and cotton gloves or socks. This helps to trap moisture in the skin and allows treatment to work more effectively.

occlusive dressings

These cover the skin closely and trap moisture. They can help treatment work more effectively on dry, thickened areas of skin.

Fingertip eczema

Some people are prone to get sore, cracked skin on the fleshy pulps and tips of their fingers. Sometimes the affected skin peels away, leaving delicate skin exposed. At other times the skin gets harder and sufferers complain that they've lost the feeling in their fingers. The fact that this site is so sensitive and important for doing fine tasks means that minor amounts of eczema here can be a great nuisance. There are different causes of fingertip eczema including allergic and irritant contact eczema. However, some adults get this problem without any obvious external cause. It may be aggravated by mild but repeated friction such as handling large quantities of paper. If you are affected, try to avoid the temptation to peel and pick away hard skin as this can cause more hard skin and cracks to develop. This is often a stubborn problem, but it can be helped by frequent use of a moisturizer, avoiding soaps or detergents, and using steroid ointments to settle any irritation.

Venous (stasis) eczema

In people with varicose veins, the blood pressure in the lower leg veins is increased (**venous hypertension**) and this has a knock-on effect on the skin here. Instead of being soft, it turns woody hard with a rusty brown discolouration, and meshes of blue-purple thread veins can be seen around the sides of the feet. These changes can occur even with mild varicose veins and may also follow a deep vein thrombosis. Eczema may develop around the inner calves and ankles, and this is called variously 'gravitational eczema', 'varicose eczema', '**venous eczema**' or 'stasis eczema'. It is most

venous hypertension
Raised pressure of blood in the veins of the lower legs.

venous eczema
Eczema on the lower legs around the ankles which is due to underlying varicose or blocked veins.

common in elderly women, but can occasionally affect younger adults. Sometimes one leg is affected much more than the other. Venous eczema is usually itchy, sore and uncomfortable, and tends to be a chronic form of eczema, although with correct treatment some cases can be cleared (see Colour Plate 12).

How should venous eczema be treated?

Venous eczema may improve if the underlying varicose veins are treated surgically. However, not everyone is suitable for an operation. Venous eczema usually responds to routine eczema treatment with moisturizers and topical steroids (see Chapter 6). It is important to keep things simple because the skin in venous eczema has an increased tendency to develop allergies to things which are applied here, including moisturizers, antibiotics, and rubber chemicals in elasticated bandages and stockings. If someone with venous eczema develops an allergy to the creams they are using, the eczema will worsen and may spread to the arms and body. It is therefore important to only apply topical treatments that are very unlikely to cause allergic reactions. Greasy ointments such as mixtures of equal parts of liquid paraffin and white soft paraffin (50/50 mix) or emulsifying ointment can be used to moisturize the skin, and topical steroids should be used in the form of ointments rather than creams as the former contain fewer additives. If someone's venous eczema does not improve with treatment or is proving difficult to control, patch tests should be considered to make sure there are no contact allergies (see Chapter 5).

Q My elderly mum has had problems with varicose leg ulcers near her ankles for several years. At the moment they are improving with special bandages that the district nurses apply, but the skin around the ulcers has become very itchy and sore, and her doctor has diagnosed eczema. How should eczema be treated when it is near a leg ulcer?

leg ulcers
These are non-healing wounds on the lower legs which may be caused by circulatory problems. Venous leg ulcers occur because of raised pressure and sluggish blood flow in the veins.

A Varicose or venous leg ulcers usually affect the skin around the lower calves above the ankles. They are often surrounded by varicose eczema. Unfortunately, skin on the lower legs heals more slowly than elsewhere, and leg ulcers sometimes prove to be a chronic problem. If they are weeping, the surface moisture can irritate the surrounding skin and aggravate eczema, and a high absorbency dressing should be used. Compression bandages or stockings are the most effective way of healing venous leg ulcers. Eczema around ulcers can be treated in the same way as venous eczema elsewhere on the leg, and treatment applied before the leg is bandaged. Topical steroids should not be applied to the ulcer itself as they may slow healing. If there are signs that the leg ulcer and surrounding skin are infected (redness, heat, swelling and leakage of unpleasant-smelling yellow-green fluid), it may be helpful to take a skin swab for bacterial testing (see Chapter 2, page 47). Infected leg ulcers should be treated with oral antibiotics or antiseptics rather than topical antibiotics as these tend to cause allergic contact eczema. Regular bathing or showering between dressing changes helps to remove surface crusting and scaling, and a simple emollient such as emulsifying ointment should be used instead of soap for washing.

Asteatotic/wintertime dry eczema

Asteatotic eczema is caused by a reduction in the skin's natural oils. Certain body sites have few grease glands, and when these become less active in older age the result is dry, cracked, sore skin. The low humidity and cold weather of winter combined with central heating or sitting close to fires or radiators make the skin drier, and this is made even worse by using soaps, shower gels and bubble baths.

Asteatotic eczema mainly affects the lower legs, arms and hands, and sometimes parts of the torso. The shins are a particular trouble zone, and often develop a crazy paving or shattered glass pattern of eczema with many fine red cracks and a dry, scaly surface. The problem is commonest in the elderly, but younger adults are occasionally affected. There is usually no underlying health problem but, rarely, generalized dryness of the skin can be due to nutritional deficiencies or an under-active thyroid gland. The most important aspect of treatment is to use plenty of greasy moisturizers and moisturizing soap substitutes. Sometimes a mild steroid ointment may be needed to settle the irritation.

Lichen simplex

Lichen simplex is an irresistibly itchy complaint that appears as a stubborn, thickened patch of eczema. The initial cause is often obscure, but once started a cycle of itching and scratching is set up which can be extremely difficult to break, and it keeps the condition going. It can affect people of all ages, and common trouble sites include the outer calves, ankles, elbows and neck (see Colour Plate 13). The genital area, especially around the anus and the scrotum or outer vulval lips (labia majora) are sometimes affected and can cause particular embarrassment. Affected areas of skin become thicker (lichenified) and darker from repeated rubbing. Sufferers are often unaware that they are scratching, especially when they are warm and sleepy in bed at night. The most important aspect of treating lichen simplex is to break the itch– scratch cycle. As people often scratch more when they feel stressed or anxious, this complaint is sometimes referred to as 'neurodermatitis'. Anti-itch creams, moisturizers and strong topical steroids may reduce the irritation, but the key to curing this complaint is to stop scratching.

CHAPTER

4

Contact eczema

Contact (exogenous) eczema, or contact dermatitis as it is more commonly called, is caused by something in the outside world that has come into direct contact with the skin. There are two main types:

1 Irritant contact eczema – due to harsh substances, usually chemical irritants.
2 Allergic contact eczema – due to substances called allergens which can be manmade or natural.

If the skin does not come into contact with the offending substances again, the eczema should get better and may clear completely. It is important to make a correct diagnosis of contact eczema because, unless the external causes are identified, the sufferer may continue to come into contact with them, and the problem will persist.

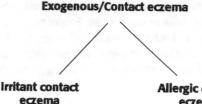

Figure 4.1 Types of exogenous eczema.

Irritant contact eczema

What is irritant contact eczema and what causes it?

Irritant contact eczema (dermatitis) occurs when the epidermis (outer skin layer) is damaged by an external substance – the irritant. Irritant chemicals are harsh substances that can harm the skin. Damage to the outer epidermal cells triggers an inflammatory reaction in the dermis, and starts an eczema reaction. If the skin is only exposed to the irritant once or intermittently, it has a chance to heal. However, if exposure is repeated and more damage occurs before healing has taken place, a chronic persistent eczema can develop.

Many different substances are **skin irritants**, ranging from mild irritants such as soap and detergents through to stronger irritants such as industrial chemicals. Although most people appreciate that strong chemicals such as solvents, acids or alkalis are harmful, milder irritants actually cause more problems and are often overlooked. Exposure to a mild irritant such as bubble bath or a shaving gel may need to be repeated many times before the damaging effects are noticeable, leaving the sufferer unaware of the underlying cause. A single or occasional exposure to a mild irritant does not usually cause any visible skin damage or symptoms. For example, most people

skin irritant
A harsh substance that can damage the skin. Irritants are classified as strong or weak irritants depending on how harmful they are.

myth
Most cases of eczema are caused by allergies.

fact
Most people with eczema have a constitutional or inbuilt tendency to get this complaint, and it is not caused by allergies. Irritant contact eczema is the commonest type of eczema with an external cause, and is much commoner than allergic contact eczema, although fewer people are aware of it.

with normal skin have no problems from washing the dishes once or twice a day. However, if they work as a kitchen cleaner and repeatedly immerse their hands in water and detergents, this is likely to damage the skin and can cause irritant contact eczema.

Q | **Who gets irritant contact eczema (dermatitis)?**

A Irritant contact eczema is most common in working age adults, and mainly affects the hands because they get the most exposure to irritants. Mothers with young babies often get irritant hand eczema for the first time because they wash their hands so frequently: after each nappy change, when washing bottles and keeping kitchen surfaces clean. People in certain occupations are more likely to suffer from irritant eczema than others because their work involves exposure to irritant substances. High-risk jobs include catering, cleaning, nursing, hairdressing and heavy industry. For example, an office worker is much less likely to get this problem than someone who works in a kitchen or factory. Some hobbies also put the skin at risk of irritation, including gardening and DIY or arts and crafts, because they involve exposure to chemicals and hand washing afterwards. Cold dry weather also acts like a skin irritant, which is why irritant hand eczema tends to be worse in the wintertime (see Colour Plate 14).

my experience

I've never had problems with my skin although my hands sometimes get dry in the winter. However, after the birth of my second baby, my hands became extremely dry and sore. This started between my fingers and under my rings, then spread over my hands, and the skin felt rough, almost like sandpaper. As my first child was still in nappies, it meant I was washing my hands almost every hour as well as cleaning up a lot of sticky food around the high chair. Putting my hands in hot water felt soothing, but seemed to make them even drier afterwards, and my skin looked wrinkled and old. Things got so bad that I was having difficulty preparing food, and my hands were really sore if I peeled fruit or vegetables.

I visited my doctor who said I had an irritant eczema (dermatitis), and prescribed a large tube of moisturizer to use whenever my skin felt dry, and she asked me to stop using soap. I kept a tub of aqueous cream by the kitchen sink and in the bathroom, and used this for washing my hands. I'd reapply my moisturizers whenever I had a few spare minutes. Wearing gloves whenever I used kitchen or bathroom cleaning chemicals meant that these did not irritate my skin anymore. I was also prescribed a steroid ointment to apply to any sore, red areas of skin at night, and to stop this making the bedclothes greasy I'd put on a pair of soft cotton gloves. After a few weeks my skin felt a lot more comfortable and the dryness and redness had faded. Six months later, when my older child was potty trained, my skin was almost back to normal. My hands can flare-up again if I don't look after them properly, but I've got things under good control most of the time.

Occasionally, other delicate body areas such as the face and axillae (underarms) can be affected by irritant contact eczema from cosmetics or toiletries. Infantile nappy rash in babies is an example of irritant contact eczema, and is caused by the repeated exposure of delicate skin to wet nappies. Irritant contact eczema is uncommon in children and the elderly because they get very little exposure to irritants.

Although irritants can damage everyone's skin, some people have more problems than others. People who have atopic eczema, or have suffered with this in the past, are more susceptible to getting irritant contact eczema.

> **Q** I've always suffered with sensitive, dry skin on my face. I've recently tried using anti-ageing eye creams, but these seem to make my skin even drier and more sore. Why does this happen?
>
> **A** Some cosmetics can irritate the delicate skin on the face, in particular the eyelids, and repeated use can cause irritant contact eczema with tight feeling skin that is dry and flaky. Skin cleansers, toners and liquid foundation often cause problems for eczema sufferers and people with sensitive skins. Anti-ageing preparations such as those containing fruit acids or vitamin A derivatives (retinoids) can be especially harsh. Avoid gels or lotions on your face, as these tend to be drying, and choose a non-fragranced thicker cream to moisturize dry areas. Do not use exfoliating products on eczema because they will remove protective outer skin layers and cause irritation.

What does irritant contact eczema look like?

Irritant contact eczema on the hands often starts as dryness and soreness or chapping, especially between the fingers, on the back of the hands (see Colour Plate 14) and under rings. It is less common on the palms where the skin is tougher. The skin feels rough, and may become cracked and red. Irritant contact eczema is much drier than other kinds of eczema, and does not usually blister or weep unless it has been caused by a very strong chemical or is infected.

> **Q** I get a lot of trouble with rashes under my arms from deodorants and antiperspirants. Some seem to cause more trouble than others, but I can't work out what's causing the problem.
>
> **A** Antiperspirants and deodorants can irritate the delicate skin in the axillae and sometimes cause eczema (dermatitis), especially if they are applied to broken skin after shaving. Strong

antiperspirants containing aluminium chloride are particularly irritating, and many people are unable to tolerate them. Deodorants also contain fragrance or perfume, and this is a common cause of allergic contact eczema. If you think you could be allergic to fragrance, try a fragrance-free antiperspirant. This should not have the word 'parfum' on the ingredient label.

How is irritant contact eczema treated?

It is important to identify which irritants have caused the problem, and to minimize contact with these. Irritant contact eczema weakens the skin barrier, so sufferers have to be more careful than usual about how they treat their skin. Exposure to all irritants should be avoided and soothing emollients applied regularly to help repair the skin. A topical steroid may be needed if there is a lot of inflammation and irritation. The skin will not have recovered completely until several weeks after it looks better, so continued care and emollients are needed.

Tips on treating irritant hand eczema

⬧ Take every opportunity to apply moisturizers. Carry a tube of cream in your pocket or handbag. Find a spare moment to reapply it whenever the skin feels rough or dry, for example, while sitting on the train or watching TV.

⬧ Avoid all soaps, detergents and liquid hand cleansers. Many simple emollients can be used as soap substitutes, and some come in pump-action dispensers which are handy to keep near the wash basins at home and at work (see Chapter 6).

⬧ Keep on being kind to your skin. Remember that the skin is vulnerable for weeks after it looks normal again.

Work-related (occupational) irritant contact eczema

Irritant contact eczema is the most common work-related skin condition. In certain jobs it is impossible to avoid all exposure to irritants, but changing tasks may reduce exposure, and protective gloves and barrier creams can help. Unfortunately these measures do not always clear the skin, and irritant contact eczema can become such a persistent problem that the person needs to change their career.

my experience

I left school at the age of 17 and had my heart set on a career in hairdressing. I'd already done a Saturday job, and started full time as a salon trainee. A few months later I started to get a rash on the back of my hands. At first it simply looked like dry skin and chapping. It got a lot better when I went on a sunny holiday, but it came back a few days after I returned to work. One of the stylists thought it was dermatitis and told me she'd had something similar when she was training. She gave me a moisturizer which helped a little, but things got much worse during the winter, and my hands became so uncomfortable that I was finding it difficult to wash clients' hair.

Thankfully, the salon manager was understanding, and let me do some reception work for a while. I visited my doctor who prescribed a steroid ointment and an emollient for moisturizing and to use instead of soap. I kept a tube of moisturizer with me and applied it during each of my breaks. When I started shampooing again, I was very careful about wearing gloves each time my hands were in water. I got a few pairs of hypoallergenic PVC gloves and also wore these when I did housework or washing-up. All this seemed to help and my hands slowly got better. I've now moved on to styling which is kinder to my skin. I still get dry, itchy hands from time to time but I now know how to cope with this and will complete my training soon.

Loss of time at work because of eczema has major financial consequences for the affected person as well as their employer, and people with suspected work-related skin conditions should be referred to a specialist in work-related diseases (occupational physician) or a dermatologist for further advice.

Allergic contact eczema

Allergic contact eczema (dermatitis) is caused by an external substance – the allergen – coming into contact with the skin of someone who is allergic to this particular substance. The allergen itself is not usually harmful, but the skin's immune system gets confused, and 'attacks' the allergen as if it were fighting an infection. The allergen does not have any effect on someone who is not allergic or sensitized to it, and it is possible to develop an allergy after many years of trouble-free contact with the allergen. In fact, someone rarely becomes allergic to an allergen if they have only been in contact with it a few times. Most everyday allergens only trigger allergies after repeated exposure.

Allergic contact eczema is a **delayed type** of **allergy**. This is a slow process, and symptoms do not start until several hours or days after skin contact with the allergen. This is a completely different process from an immediate allergy reaction like hay fever (see Chapter 5, page 88). Because of this time ·lag, people can easily overlook a delayed allergy, and it can be very difficult to work out what is causing the problem, even if an allergy is suspected. For example, if someone develops a rash on their neck on a Tuesday morning, they may not realize it has been caused by an allergy to the aftershave they wore on Saturday night.

> **delayed type allergy**
> An allergy reaction that starts hours or days after exposure to the allergen.

fact

Natural products such as essential oils from plants and lanolin from sheep's wool are well-known allergens, and are among the most common causes of allergic contact eczema. Because of this, scientists are trying to create synthetic fragrances that smell like natural fragrances but are less likely to cause allergic reactions.

What are the commonest causes of allergic contact eczema?

Thousands of substances have been reported to cause allergic contact eczema, but most reactions are caused by a limited number of allergens. The following are the most common culprits:

◇ Nickel in metal jewellery, belt buckles and eyeglass frames

◇ Perfumes in fine fragrances, cosmetics and toiletries

◇ Rubber chemicals in household gloves and footwear

◇ Chemical hair dye

◇ Preservative chemicals in cosmetics and toiletries

◇ Chromate which is used in the tanning of leather and in cement

◇ Plants in the house and garden, and plant extracts in cosmetics

◇ Ingredients in topical medicaments and moisturizers.

fact

These products can still contain allergens and can therefore cause allergic contact eczema. The term 'hypoallergenic' usually means that a common allergen such as fragrance (perfume) is not present in a cosmetic or toiletry, but other allergens may still be present and cause problems if you are allergic to them.

Q Is allergic contact eczema caused by something I am eating or by a food allergy?

A Allergic contact eczema is caused by something external that comes into contact with the skin, and it is not caused by food or anything taken by mouth. The only rare exception to this rule is among people who handle food and get an allergic contact eczema from food on their hands.

What does allergic contact eczema look like?

Skin affected with allergic contact eczema is red, swollen, flaky and itchy, just like other kinds of eczema (see Colour Plate 15). As a result of this similarity, the diagnosis may not be suspected, especially if someone already has a constitutional or endogenous type of eczema (see Chapter 1). It is therefore important to consider the possibility of contact allergy if eczema occurs in an unusual pattern or fails to improve with appropriate treatment. Allergic contact eczema can affect people of all ages, but is very uncommon in babies and young children, because their skin has only had limited exposure to contact allergens. Allergic contact eczema affects the area of skin that has been in contact with the allergen. The rash is usually localized, but if there is a strong allergy it may spread to the surrounding skin. Allergic contact eczema mainly affects body areas that have most contact with allergens. These include the following:

◇ Hands and feet
◇ Face
◇ Axillae (underarms)
◇ Lower legs with venous eczema (see Chapter 3).

How is allergic contact eczema treated?

The treatment of allergic contact eczema involves three important steps:

1 Treat the eczema with topical steroids and emollients (see Chapter 6).
2 Identify the allergen(s) by patch testing (see Chapter 5).
3 Avoid future exposure to these allergens.

my experience

I've had pierced ears since my teens and have always been careful to wear gold or silver earrings as cheaper earrings make my ears crusty and sore, even if I only wear them for a few hours. Several of my friends have the same sort of problem, so I think this is quite common. However, when I got a sore rash below my belly button, I did not guess that this was being caused by the metal in my belt buckle. The rash got very sore and looked infected, so I saw my doctor who prescribed a strong steroid cream with antibiotics. He suspected that the rash was caused by a nickel allergy and asked me to stop wearing the belt. I did, and after a week the rash was much better, although the eczema left a dark patch of skin for a few months. I tried wearing the belt again, and after a few days the rash started to come back, which proved to me that it had caused the problem.

Allergic contact eczema can be extremely itchy and uncomfortable, and it needs active treatment with topical steroids and simple emollients. The ingredients of moisturizers and medicaments can cause allergies, and so it is best to choose products that contain the fewest possible allergens, for example 50:50 liquid paraffin/ white soft paraffin and a steroid ointment rather than cream, because creams contain preservatives.

Patch testing is usually needed to find or confirm which allergen(s) could be causing the eczema. Once the culprit has been identified, it is important to try and avoid future skin contact with this allergen. If this is achieved, and someone does not have any underlying eczema, there is an excellent chance that the eczema will clear completely. Once a contact allergy has developed, it tends to be life-long, so continued care is needed to avoid the allergen(s). People who are allergic to ingredients of cosmetics and toiletries need to read the ingredient labels carefully in order to avoid using a product that contains these allergens. Unfortunately, for some other allergies such as household and industrial chemicals or shoe components, it is much more difficult to find out what can be used safely. The main things to remember are:

✧ Allergic contact eczema is caused by skin contact with an allergen in someone who is allergic to this substance.

✧ An allergy may develop after many years of trouble-free contact with the allergen.

✧ Allergic contact eczema is a slow (delayed type) allergy process, which takes several hours or days to appear and many days to clear.

✧ Allergic contact eczema is not caused by anything you have eaten.

my experience

I'm 55 years old and I had been using hair dyes for over ten years without any problems. However, six months ago I developed an itchy sore rash on the back of my neck and forehead. I tried changing my shampoo, which did not help, and saw my doctor who diagnosed eczema and gave me a steroid cream. The rash seemed to get worse the day after I dyed my hair, whether I did it at home or in a salon. Because the eczema did not clear, I was referred to a dermatologist and she arranged patch tests to see if it was being caused by an allergy. I was very surprised when these showed that I had become allergic to chemical hair dye. I thought you could not become allergic to something you had used for so long, but the dermatologist explained that, in fact, the opposite was true and that allergies could start after years of safely using a product! She also explained that this sort of allergy was usually life-long. I was quite upset about the thought of not being able to use hair dye again, but have now got used to the idea of being glamorous and grey and am pleased to report that my rash has gone away.

Q My five-year-old son has atopic eczema. He's been given many different creams and ointments but when his skin is bad he complains that these sting or burn within a few minutes of being applied. They seem to make him scratch and the eczema becomes red and sore. Is this an allergy and should he have tests?

A Many eczema sufferers notice that their skin itches or stings within minutes of applying certain creams. This does not mean that they are allergic to this product, but rather that their skin is very sensitive and easily irritated. This happens because the product is being applied to skin that is already upset and damaged. It's a little like the stinging sensation you get if lemon juice gets into a cut. This is not an allergy; allergic contact eczema happens much more slowly over several hours or days, so allergy tests are not needed.

Unfortunately, no moisturizer can be guaranteed not to sting. Ointments tend to sting less than creams, and fragrance should be avoided as it can cause irritation.

My elderly mum has had a lot of trouble with her legs for more than ten years. She has had stubborn varicose ulcers that have now thankfully healed, but her skin is discoloured with redness and dryness around the upper inner ankle area. She has tried many different moisturizers, some on prescription, and others bought from the local supermarket. Over the last six months her rash flared up and spread up to her knees. Because it was so itchy, she tried all sorts of creams, but nothing helped. Her doctor diagnosed varicose eczema and prescribed a strong steroid cream that helped. However, one weekend her skin became much worse and the rash spread on to her body and arms. She was really upset and uncomfortable, so the doctor arranged an urgent appointment at the hospital. She saw a dermatologist who stopped all her old creams, and prescribed a simple emulsifying ointment for moisturizing and washing, and another steroid ointment. They also gave her a week's treatment with antibiotics as the eczema on her legs looked weepy and infected. This seemed to work quite well and her eczema settled down again. When her skin was better, she had patch tests. These showed that my mum was allergic to lanolin in one of her favourite moisturizers, and an antibiotic called neomycin in a steroid cream that she'd been given, and pine resin or colophony which is present in old-fashioned sticking plasters, although she hadn't used these for years. They concluded that she had developed an allergy to her creams on top of her underlying venous eczema.

My mum is now very careful about what she puts on her skin, and avoids anything which contains the substances she is allergic to. This seems to be keeping her eczema under good control although it has not gone away.

CHAPTER

5

Allergy tests in eczema

There are two important types of allergy reaction in the skin: immediate and delayed. Immediate allergy reactions cause a red bumpy rash called **'hives'** or **'urticaria'** (nettle rash), which appears within minutes of exposure to allergens, and settles after an hour or so. Delayed allergy reactions appear as an eczema (see Chapter 4, page 81) and develop slowly over hours or days after exposure to the allergen; they also last for several days. Immediate and delayed type allergy rashes differ in their appearance and duration because they involve different allergy mechanisms. Consequently, the allergy tests used to investigate them are not the same.

Immediate type allergy reactions are usually investigated with skin prick tests and blood tests to measure IgE antibody levels, whereas delayed type allergy (or allergic contact eczema) is investigated with patch tests. These tests are explained in more detail below.

> **hives or urticaria**
> This is an itchy, bumpy, swollen rash which looks like a nettle rash.

Tests for immediate allergy reactions

What happens in an immediate allergy reaction?

The symptoms of immediate allergy include itchy, watery eyes (conjunctivitis), a runny nose with sneezing (rhinitis), wheezing (asthma), and a bumpy red rash called 'hives' or 'urticaria' (nettle rash). In severe cases, allergy reactions can lead to collapse and anaphylactic shock. The reaction occurs because the allergic person has developed IgE antibodies against the allergen. These antibodies are attached to special cells in the eyes, nose, airways and skin called 'mast cells'. When the allergy sufferer is exposed to the allergen, it binds to the IgE antibodies, and this triggers the mast cells to release histamine and other chemicals which then causes the symptoms mentioned above. The precise symptoms and severity depend on how much allergen has come into contact with the body and how allergic someone is. IgE antibodies can be measured in a blood sample and demonstrated by skin prick tests.

Immediate type allergy tests have a limited role in eczema management. They may be indicated in childhood atopic eczema to investigate food allergies (see Chapter 2, page 43), and to investigate sensitivity to airborne allergens (house dust mites, animal fur and pollens) in all ages. People who have hand eczema and symptoms of itching or redness on wearing rubber gloves should also be investigated with immediate allergy tests for natural rubber latex allergy, as this can cause severe reactions as well as aggravating eczema (see Chapter 3, page 61).

It is important to appreciate that immediate allergy tests only identify allergens which could act as an aggravating factor in eczema; they do not unearth its cause.

What are skin prick tests?

Skin prick tests are a quick and reliable way of investigating if a person is sensitized to an allergen. However, the story becomes a little complicated here because some people react to allergens on prick testing, but do not seem to have any problem when they encounter these allergens in daily life. They are said to be 'sensitized', but not 'symptomatic'. It is possible that with time these people will develop allergy symptoms, but there seem to be mechanisms in the body that can hold them at bay. Prick testing therefore shows which allergens the patient may be allergic to, but does not tell us whether these allergies are causing or contributing to their symptoms. This is why it is so important for the doctor to take a detailed history in order to interpret the allergy test results properly.

Prick tests are usually carried out on the inner forearm or back. Small drops of allergen solution are pricked into the outermost layers of the skin with a fine needle or lancet. The needle prick is slightly uncomfortable, but no worse than having a hair plucked. When someone is allergic to an allergen, they develop a small, red, itchy swelling or wheal where it has been applied which looks like an insect bite. The wheal usually develops within ten minutes and disappears within an hour. This means that prick tests give an almost immediate visual result that the patient and doctor can discuss (see Colour Plate 16).

skin prick tests
Tests carried out on the skin to demonstrate immediate type allergies.

Prick testing to airborne allergens, such as pollens, animal fur and house dust mite, is extremely safe. Testing to other substances such as food and drugs carries a small risk of triggering severe allergy reactions, so resuscitation facilities should always be available. These tests can be carried out on people of all ages, including young children, but cannot be done if there is widespread eczema. Antihistamines should be stopped several days before prick tests as they may prevent allergy reactions from showing up.

What are allergy blood tests?

The levels of IgE antibodies that react to allergens that cause immediate type reactions can be measured in a blood sample. These tests are most commonly called RAST or immuno CAP® tests. They are carried out in a laboratory, and the results may take several weeks. One advantage of blood tests is that IgE antibodies to many different allergens can be measured from one sample. The results are graded from 0–6 where 0 means no detectable IgE against the allergen (which means that an allergy is very unlikely) and 6 means a high level of IgE (allergy very likely). The problem with allergy blood tests is that they often pick up low levels of antibodies that are not causing symptoms. These are called 'false positive results' and they happen most in people who have quite severe atopic conditions (eczema, asthma and hay fever). False positive results are especially common to foods, so people with severe eczema may end up with a list of 'allergies' to foods they are actually able to eat without any problem. Rather than solving any question, extensive food allergy tests like these often cause confusion and anxiety. The tests are simple, but skill and expertise is needed in order to interpret them properly and decide which allergens need to be avoided.

Children with eczema should never be put on exclusion diets on the basis of food allergy blood tests without medical advice and dietary supervision (see Chapter 2, page 41).

Other sorts of test for immediate allergies

It may sometimes be necessary to carry out a challenge test to investigate immediate type allergies, for example when someone has a history that strongly suggests an immediate allergy, but prick tests or blood test results are negative. In order to clarify whether they are really allergic or not, a challenge test can be performed whereby the allergen is given in very small quantities by mouth or injected into the skin. This sort of testing is mainly used for drug allergies and food allergies. It can cause severe allergic reactions and should only be done in specialized clinics by trained staff.

Tests for delayed allergy reactions

Patch tests

Patch tests have been carried out for over 100 years to diagnose allergic contact eczema. They are extremely safe and simple but are quite time-consuming and require medical and nursing expertise as well as facilities to store the allergens correctly. The tests are usually done on the skin of

myth
Alternative allergy tests such as vega testing and kinaesthesiology can identify food allergies and are helpful in eczema.

fact
These and other tests such as hair analysis are not recommended as there is no scientific evidence that they reliably identify allergies of any kind.

patch tests
Skin allergy tests to investigate possible allergic contact eczema.

the upper back because this area is quite flat and relatively undisturbed by movement. They can also be done on the upper arms and chest. The test allergens should only be applied to skin that looks normal and is not affected by eczema, otherwise the results are difficult to interpret.

Small quantities of allergens are placed against the skin in small discs on large sticky pieces of tape – the patches. These need to be stuck closely onto the body to allow the allergens to be absorbed into the skin. The patches are removed after two days, and the skin is inspected to see if any allergens have caused an area of eczema. It may take several days for this to appear. Many dermatologists will carry out two skin inspections, firstly two days after the patches were applied and secondly four days afterwards. Sometimes the skin reactions appear so slowly that it is necessary to re-examine the skin a week after the patches were applied.

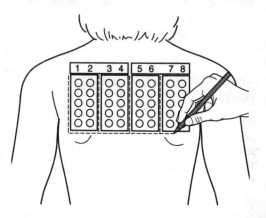

Figure 5.1 Patch tests on the upper back.

An allergic patch test reaction appears as a small itchy patch of swollen, red skin about the size of a fingernail. In strong allergic reactions, the skin may also blister and weep. Someone who is not allergic to the test allergens will not get any rash. The allergens are placed in a precise order and the patches are outlined in ink so the doctor can tell which allergen has caused the reaction. This means that the test area cannot be washed until the tests are completed.

Q Why are the tests done on my back when my eczema has never affected this part of my body?

A If someone is allergic to an allergen, they will get a rash on any body area where the allergen comes into contact. For example, if you are allergic to perfume, you will get the same sort of rash wherever it is applied to the skin. The upper back is the ideal place for patch tests as the body surface here is quite flat and broad, allowing the patches and allergens to stay close against the skin, which helps them to work better.

Q Are there any forms of medication or treatment that can interfere with the results of patch tests?

A Thankfully few things affect the results of patch tests. If someone is taking high doses of steroid tablets these can reduce or prevent allergies from showing up. Sunbathing can also reduce patch test reactions, making the results less reliable. So, the tests should not be carried out if someone has a suntan or is receiving ultraviolet treatment for their eczema.

myth
You can't take antihistamine tablets if you are having patch tests.

fact
Patch tests detect slow or delayed type allergy reactions which do not involve the chemical histamine. The results are therefore not affected by antihistamine medication, but can be suppressed if someone is taking a high dose of steroid tablets by mouth. This is different from prick tests, where antihistamines should be stopped several days beforehand.

Q **Can patch tests be carried out during pregnancy?**

A Although there is no evidence that they can cause harm to the developing baby, patch testing is not recommended during pregnancy. This is because of the theoretical risk that the baby could be affected by the allergens which are applied to the mother's skin.

At the end of the tests, the dermatologist will explain the results to the patient and advise how to avoid any allergens that they are allergic to. Patch testing allows the skin to be tested to many different allergens at one time and is extremely safe.

What allergens are applied to the skin?

The allergens which are routinely tested are those that commonly cause allergic contact eczema (see Chapter 4, page 81). These include fragrances, metals, rubber chemicals, plant derivatives, and the ingredients of medicated creams, cosmetics and toiletries. People who are exposed to different chemicals through their work or hobbies may need to be tested with additional allergens, for example, photographic colour developers, hairdressing chemicals, metalworking fluids. Patch test allergens are bought from specialist manufacturers who purify and prepare them at a specific concentration to avoid irritating the skin. Sometimes it is necessary to test people with their own creams, cosmetics, clothes and work chemicals.

Other sorts of test for delayed allergies

If a skincare product such as a body lotion seems to have caused a rash it can be helpful to carry out a 'use' or 'repeat open application' test. This involves applying the lotion to a small area in your

myth
Patch tests are used to diagnose food allergies.

fact
Patch tests can help diagnose allergies to substances in the outside world which come into contact with the skin. They are not used for the investigation or diagnosis of dietary allergies.

elbow crease every morning and night for up to a week. If redness and itchy bumps appear, this suggests you may be allergic to something in the product. This type of test can be a simple way of testing for a cosmetic or medicament allergy, but it should not be done with products that are not usually left on the skin such as a shampoo or rinse-off cleansers.

my experience

I recently developed a sore rash around my underarms which spread on to my face and upper neck. My doctor diagnosed eczema and gave me some steroid creams. When the rash did not clear up, he referred me to a dermatologist for patch tests to see if I was allergic to something.

The patch tests were carried out in the outpatient department. I was asked to bring along anything I'd been putting on the rash, including moisturizers, prescribed creams and toiletries. I had to remove the clothes on my upper body, except my bra, and a nurse applied five large patches on my upper back. They looked like large, white sticking plasters, and each patch had rows of tiny metal discs that contained the test allergens.

The nurse drew an ink outline around the patches and explained that I needed to keep them in place for two days. She said it was important that they stayed in close contact with the skin and asked me to keep as cool and dry as possible. The patches felt odd and slightly uncomfortable at first, but they did not hurt. I cancelled my yoga class and could not shower, but was able to take a shallow bath without getting my back wet. I took more time getting dressed and undressed, because raising my arms seemed to make the patches move. I went back to the hospital two days later, and the patches were taken off. The doctor examined my back to see if there had been any reactions. I noticed some discoloured areas and several small, red, itchy areas. I had to keep my back dry for another two days, then returned for my third visit to the clinic. My back was re-examined and the doctor told me that I was allergic to fragrances. I had reacted to the mixture of fragrances they use routinely in the tests as well as to my own deodorant and a body lotion. The doctor said this was likely to have been the cause of my eczema and explained how to avoid products containing fragrance in the future.

myth
Everyone with eczema should have allergy tests to find the cause.

fact
Most types of eczema are inbuilt or endogenous, in which case there is no underlying allergy, and these tests will not provide any helpful information. Patch tests are only needed when there is a suspicion that someone has allergic contact eczema. There are no hard and fast rules about this, but allergic contact eczema is more likely if the eczema affects certain body areas or gets worse or fails to respond to topical treatment.

It felt good to have a long soak in the bath that evening. I spent some time going through my bathroom cabinet and threw out all the toiletries which had the word 'parfum' on the label. I was surprised just how many there were. I've bought a fragrance-free antiperspirant and my skin is a lot better. I miss wearing perfume but it's worth it not to get rashes again.

CHAPTER

6

Eczema treatment

The aims of eczema treatment are to soothe and control the condition. This will in turn reduce the irritation and soreness that can cause so much discomfort and disturbance in daily life. For most sufferers, there is no cure that clears eczema permanently, but it is important to keep a positive attitude about treatment as there is now more choice than ever before, and most people with eczema will be able to manage their skin with relatively simple and safe therapy.

Topical treatment

A **topical treatment** is something that is applied to the surface of the skin rather than taken internally. The two most commonly used topical treatments for eczema are emollients or moisturizers and steroids.

> **topical treatment**
> A treatment that is applied to the surface of the body rather than being taken internally.

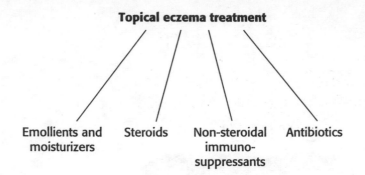

Figure 6.1 Topical eczema treatment.

Most eczema sufferers will be able to keep their eczema under control by using these treatments correctly. Other topical treatments for eczema include antibiotics to treat non-steroidal infections and the newer immunosuppressants.

Emollients and moisturizers

emollients and moisturizers
Soothing preparations that help the skin retain moisture and improve dryness.

The term **'emollient'** literally means a soothing, calming substance. This name refers to simple moisturizers for use on eczema and other skin complaints, rather than cosmetic moisturizers which contain many more ingredients and additives. Most people use the terms **'emollient'** and **'moisturizer'** interchangeably, but strictly speaking an emollient simply acts as a barrier to prevent loss of the skin's own moisture while a moisturizer has additional humectants – substances that increase the water content of the skin.

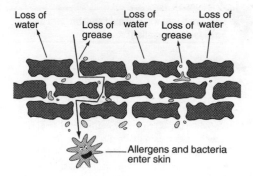

a) Skin affected by eczema

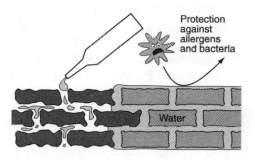

b) Eczema treatment with emollients.

Figure 6.2 (a) Skin cells in eczema lose moisture and shrivel. Surface cracks allow allergens and bacteria to penetrate into skin;
(b) Emollients increase skin moisture levels and restore the skin barrier so it can protect against allergens and infection.

A   Emollients and moisturizers should be applied to eczema frequently and freely, whenever the skin feels dry. They soak in best after a warm bath or shower when the skin is still slightly damp. They can be dabbed over the body as small dots and should be smoothed gently in the direction of hair growth, taking care not to rub hard as this can set off itching. Pump-action dispensers may be more hygienic than a tub of emollient. Hands should be washed before applying them because putting dirty hands in tubs of cream can lead to contamination with bacteria.

How do I choose the right one?

The wide range of emollients can be rather bewildering for any newcomers with eczema. The right emollient is the one that you like, so choose small pots or tubes first and see which you prefer. You may need several different emollients, for example, a lighter cream to use during the day at school or work, and a heavier ointment after bathing and last thing at night. Emollients can be bought without prescription but it is usually less expensive in the long run to have them on a National Health Service (NHS) prescription. It is important that you are prescribed sufficient quantities. For instance, to treat widespread dry eczema, a child will require 250 g/week and an adult 500 g/week.

As a general rule, the runnier the moisturizer, the less effective it will be. Greasy preparations that stay in the pot when tipped upside down are best for dry skin. Cosmetic moisturizers are not recommended because they are not intended for use on skin complaints, and may contain irritating or allergy-provoking ingredients such as fragrances. They are usually much more expensive than simple emollients and are not available on prescription.

Q Why is soap such a bad thing for eczema?

A Soaps have a very alkaline pH, and this can upset the naturally acidic surface of the skin. Soaps are effective at removing dirt and grease, but also remove the skin's natural oils which can cause drying and a tight uncomfortable feeling. This even happens with mild soaps, liquid soaps and those with added moisturizers, so all soap should be avoided on eczema and dry skin. Simple emollient creams and ointments, such as aqueous cream or emulsifying ointment, can be used instead and will clean the skin surface without drying. Emollients in pump-action dispensers are very convenient and can be kept next to the kitchen or bathroom sink for hand washing.

One of the many possible reasons why childhood atopic eczema has increased in recent years is that we now wash much more often and use many soaps and shower gels as skin cleansers. The drying effect of soap and washing damages the skin surface and this allows the skin's own moisture to be lost by evaporation. Surface cracks also allow bacteria and microbes to enter the skin, and this can trigger eczema.

Ointments

Ointments are the greasiest of moisturizers. They do not contain water, and provide an occlusive layer that reduces the evaporation of water from the skin surface and traps moisture in the skin. Most ointments are made from mineral oils (paraffin, petroleum jelly) but some come from animal or vegetable fats or are synthetic. They are especially helpful in treating very dry skin, but can be unpopular because they make clothes and bedding greasy. Ointments are very resistant to bacterial and fungal contamination because they do not contain water, and they do not usually need antimicrobial preservatives. One of the simplest and most effective emollients is a

ointments
Greasy preparations that keep moisture in the skin and improve dry skin complaints.

mixture of equal parts (50:50) liquid paraffin and white soft paraffin. It is truly 'hypoallergenic' because it does not contain added chemicals such as fragrances or preservatives, and it is an ideal choice for eczema treatment where contact allergies are a problem. Ointments work best at trapping skin moisture when the skin is well hydrated after soaking in a warm bath.

Q   I have eczema but love to add something to my bath. Can I use moisturizing bubble baths or bath oils?

A   As a simple rule, anything that makes soapy bubbles tends to dry the skin and worsen eczema. This includes bubble baths, even those labelled as 'mild' or 'moisturizing'. If you like to add something to your bath or the children's bath, choose an emollient bath oil instead. There are several different kinds, and these can be obtained on prescription. They are pleasant to use and soothing, but can make the bath extremely slippery so special care is needed with children and the elderly. Some bath oils form a film on the surface of the water, while others disperse in the water and turn it a milky colour.

Creams

creams

Preparations containing a mixture of oil and water that are used to treat skin complaints and may act as moisturizers. They usually look white.

Creams contain a mixture of oil and water in variable proportions – oily creams containing relatively more oil than simple creams. An emulsifier needs to be added to ensure an even mixture because oil and water usually separate from one another. Once applied, the water mostly evaporates, although some may be absorbed by the outer epidermis. The most important effect is the thin film of oil left on the surface which traps moisture in the skin.

Lotions

Lotions are watery preparations that contain the least oil and are of little use in eczema, but they do have a cooling effect – hence their use in conditions like sunburn. Because they are non-greasy, they may be useful for treating hairy areas such as the scalp. Their high water content means that preservative chemicals need to be added to prevent bacterial and fungal growth.

Added ingredients

Some emollients contain added ingredients to improve their effectiveness or to give additional actions:

◇ **Humectants** are substances that increase the ability of emollients to moisturize the skin. They include natural chemicals such as urea and lactic acid which are found in sweat. They are especially useful for hard, dry skin areas but can cause stinging.

◇ **Anti-itch** ingredients (anti-pruritics) occasionally present in emollients include lauromacrogols and menthol.

◇ **Antiseptics** reduce the level of bacteria on the skin, which can aggravate eczema and trigger a flare. They include benzalkonium chloride, triclosan and chlorhexidine. These chemicals can sometimes cause irritation.

Q **When are bandages and wet wraps used for eczema treatment?**

A Children with moderate or severe eczema may benefit from covering affected areas of skin with paste bandages or wet wraps. Paste bandages are quite an old-fashioned remedy for eczema and are quite messy and time-consuming. Nevertheless, they can be especially soothing for stubborn, scratched eczema on the arms and legs.

Wet wraps consist of a damp layer of stretchy tube dressing that is applied to the skin after moisturizing and then covered with a dry layer of dressing or clothing. Wet wraps can be put on the

A arms and legs or made into a whole body suit to cover the torso. Once again they are time-consuming, and take practice – the help and expertise of a dermatology nurse practitioner is invaluable in teaching this technique to parents or carers. Wet wraps can be used during the day and at night. If the child wears them to school, special support will be needed from teachers and other school staff to help deal with comments and questions from other children. The coolness of wet wraps can be very soothing for the irritable skin of eczema, and they help to break the itch–scratch cycle. The inner layer can be remoistened with water from a mister spray, as used to water household plants. Older children and adults do not usually like wet wraps because they get too cold, so this treatment is mainly used for young children. Wet wraps and bandages should not be used when eczema looks infected because occluding the skin can worsen infection.

Topical steroids

steroids
Steroids are a group of chemicals which include natural hormones produced by the body. The steroids used to treat eczema and other inflammatory conditions are corticosteroids. These calm inflammation and reduce over-activity of the immune system.

The **steroids** used in the treatment of eczema and other inflammatory skin diseases are a group of substances called 'corticosteroids', which are related to the body's natural hormone cortisol. They should not be confused with anabolic steroids such as testosterone, which are used illegally by some athletes to build up muscles. Cortisol and other corticosteroids have many anti-inflammatory actions, which is why they are used for a variety of medical problems from asthma to arthritis. These anti-inflammatory actions include reducing skin blood flow and suppressing the influx of fighter white blood cells into the skin. They also slow the rate of growth of epidermal skin cells and dermal collagen fibres.

For most medical problems, steroids need to be taken internally, but one of the good things about treating skin complaints is that medications can work effectively when applied externally, i.e. topically. There are fewer problems from using steroids topically than when they are taken internally. In the early years of use, before doctors were aware of the side effects, strong steroids were prescribed for long-term treatment of skin complaints on delicate skin areas such as the eyelids, face and skin folds. This led to skin damage in the form of thinning (**steroid atrophy**), stretch marks (striae), 'broken veins' and persistent facial redness. However, it is now over 50 years since **topical steroids** were first used, and there is a great deal of experience in getting the best out of steroid treatment while minimizing the chances of skin damage. Unfortunately, the memory of steroid atrophy has lingered and it has created a phobia of steroids among eczema sufferers and their carers. Sometimes this anxiety leads to the eczema sufferer being denied safe effective treatment and relief of symptoms.

Topical steroids are usually very effective at suppressing mild to moderate eczema as well as other inflammatory rashes. This gives the skin a chance to heal and helps break the itch–scratch cycle that worsens eczema. However, it would be a mistake to think of steroids as a cure and eczema may come back or relapse when the treatment is stopped. This can cause frustration for eczema sufferers because it makes treatment seem like a game of snakes and ladders.

steroid atrophy
Thinning of the skin due to the use of a topical steroid or from taking high doses of steroids internally.

topical steroids
Topical steroids are a group of anti-inflammatory medicaments (corticosteroids) used topically (applied to the skin surface) in the treatment of eczema and some other skin complaints.

Q There are so many topical steroids. What's the difference between them?

A Topical steroids are grouped into four strengths:

✧ Mild
✧ Moderate
✧ Strong (potent)
✧ Very strong (super-potent).

myth
All topical steroids are dangerous and cause skin damage.

fact
Topical steroids come in four different strengths. Skin thinning is only likely when strong or very strong steroids are used long term, especially on delicate areas of skin such as the eyelids and skin folds (flexures) around the armpits and groin. Milder steroids rarely, if ever, cause this problem when used sensibly. Internal (or systemic) side effects from topical steroids are very uncommon but can occur if stronger preparations are overused. In order to prevent this, the maximum recommended weekly dose is 50 g for very potent steroids and 100 g for potent steroids.

Although topical steroids look similar, there is a world of difference between the effectiveness and safety of strong or very strong steroids and mild steroids. In general, the stronger the steroid, the more effective it is, and the more likely it is to cause unwanted effects such as skin atrophy. For this reason, only mild steroids should be used on delicate areas such as the eyelids. However, these are usually ineffective on the thick skin of the palms and soles, where a stronger steroid is needed. The choice of steroid also depends on how severe and widespread the eczema is. Small stubborn patches of very active eczema such as lichen simplex (see Chapter 3, page 72) may need a strong steroid, but a milder steroid would be used to treat a larger body area. Young children (under five years) are usually prescribed mild steroids, although occasionally they may need stronger preparations.

Like moisturizers, topical steroids come as ointments, creams and lotions that vary in their greasiness. There are also gels for hairy areas like the scalp. In general, an ointment is best for dry, scaly, cracked eczema while a cream is easier to apply to weepy acute eczema. Ointments are more moisturizing and contain fewer additives such as preservatives.

Some steroids contain additional active ingredients, including the following:

✧ Antibiotics to treat bacterial infection

✧ Antifungals to treat yeasts and fungal infections

✧ Coal tar to calm inflammation and reduce skin scaling

✧ Salicylic acid to soften thickened skin

✧ Urea to hydrate the skin.

One of the problems with tubes of steroids is that they do not have any coding to indicate their strength. It is very important that people applying topical steroids know exactly which ones to use on different body sites. If you are unsure, ask your doctor to write a simple list of what to use where, and mark the strengths on the tube packets, or speak to your pharmacist.

Q **How do I know where to apply a steroid, and how often should it be used to treat eczema?**

A Topical steroids should be applied to active areas of eczema that feel rough or raised and look red. Although they can have an immediate soothing effect on the skin, they should *not* be used as emollients. The anti-inflammatory actions of steroids take several hours, so any immediate relief they give is purely because of their cream or ointment base. Steroids should be used to treat eczema flares, and they may be more effective if started early rather than delayed a few days. If the eczema is quite severe, it is usually necessary to start with a moderate or strong steroid on the body every day for a week or two, then reduce to a milder steroid, or use the stronger preparation less frequently. Once the redness and swelling of eczema has settled, steroid treatment should be stopped, and any remaining dryness and irritation treated with emollients. Topical steroids are usually applied twice a day, but some newer preparations are effective when only used once a day.

> ### Q How much steroid should I use?
>
> **A** Topical steroids should be applied gently as a thin layer on affected skin. The 'fingertip unit' (FTU) can be a helpful guide to steroid use in eczema. A fingertip dose is the amount of steroid cream or ointment that covers the fleshy pulp of an adult finger from the crease over the first joint to the tip of the finger. The number of fingertip doses or units recommended to treat a body area vary according to the affected person's size. For example, four fingertip units treat one arm and hand in an adult, while only one fingertip unit would be needed to treat this area in a baby.

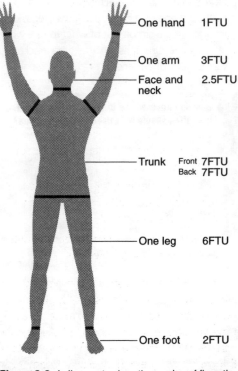

One hand	1FTU
One arm	3FTU
Face and neck	2.5FTU
Trunk	Front 7FTU
	Back 7FTU
One leg	6FTU
One foot	2FTU

Figure 6.3 A diagram to show the number of fingertip doses (units) of steroid used to treat different body areas in an adult.

myth
Because they are dangerous, steroids can only be obtained with a prescription.

fact
Some mild topical steroids (0.1, 0.5 and 1 per cent hydrocortisone) and a moderate strength topical steroid (clobetasone butyrate) are available from pharmacies in the UK without prescription. This is not medically supervised, so purchasers are advised not to use these preparations on the face or genital area, during pregnancy or on young children. This is a precaution in case the treatment was being used inapproprlately, and although it is sensible advice, it can make people feel unnecessarily worried about using topical steroids.

What to do if a steroid doesn't help

If a topical steroid does not seem to be working in eczema there are several possible reasons, including the following:

⬥ The eczema is too severe and the steroid too mild

⬥ Not enough steroid has been applied, or treatment stopped too soon – often because the eczema sufferer is afraid of side effects

⬥ The person has an allergy to an ingredient in the topical steroid or another treatment being applied to the skin

⬥ The diagnosis is wrong, for example, not eczema but a fungal infection.

On rare instances, steroids can actually cause allergic reactions. This is easily overlooked because they also have anti-inflammatory actions. However, it should be suspected if someone's eczema gets worse after applying a topical steroid. If there is any question of allergy to any topical medicament including steroids, patch tests should be carried out (see Chapter 5, page 91).

Table 2 The important differences between moisturizers and topical steroids.

	Moisturizers	Steroids
What do they do?	Trap moisture in the skin which reduces dryness and relieves discomfort and itch	Reduce inflammation (redness, heat, swelling, itch and soreness) shortly after applying
Where to apply?	To all dry skin areas and active areas of eczema	To inflamed areas of eczema − where skin is red, hot and itchy
How much?	As much as is needed to make the skin feel softer and comfortable − no limit	A thin layer smoothed into affected areas of skin
How frequently?	As often as is needed and is possible. At least twice a day, ideally more often, whenever the skin feels tight and dry − no limit	Once or twice a day only
Problems with use	◇ Can cause stinging or itching shortly after applying ◇ People may dislike the feel of greasy preparations ◇ Rarely can cause allergic eczema	◇ Can sometimes sting or itch shortly ◇ Overuse of stronger steroids, especially on delicate areas (face, flexures), can cause skin thinning, stretch marks and redness ◇ May make the rash worse if used for the wrong conditions, for example fungal infections

Topical antibiotics

The skin surface in eczema has tiny cracks, which can make it prone to infections. This is especially true of atopic eczema (see Chapters 2 and 3), but also applies to other forms of eczema such as discoid eczema, hand and foot eczema and contact eczema (see Chapters 3 and 4). For this reason, topical antibacterial or antifungal agents (antibiotics) are sometimes combined with a topical steroid. Combined preparations are especially useful at certain body sites, such as the anogenital area or the feet, where a variety of microbes can cause infections.

However, long-term use of topical antibiotics is not recommended as it encourages growth of resistant bacteria. People can also become allergic to topical antibiotics, which means that using them will actually make the eczema worse.

Non-steroidal immunosuppressants

One of the latest developments in eczema treatment is a new group of drugs called 'non-steroidal **immunosuppressants**' or 'topical calcineurin inhibitors' (TCIs). When taken internally, these drugs have a powerful damping-down or suppressant effect on the immune system, which is why they are used to prevent the rejection of transplanted organs. When applied to the skin, non-steroidal immunosuppressants reduce the overactivity of the skin's immune system that occurs in eczema. At present the two drugs of this kind which have been approved in the UK for treatment of atopic eczema are:

> **immuno-suppressant**
> An agent that reduces the activity of the body's immune system.

1. Pimecrolimus (as a cream)
2. Tacrolimus (as an ointment).

Topical tacrolimus has been found to be as effective as a potent steroid, and is more effective than pimecrolimus cream.

The major advantage of using topical non-steroidal immunosuppressants is that, unlike topical steroids, they do not cause skin thinning (atrophy). This could be especially useful when treating eczema on thin areas of skin such as the eyelids, face and neck.

Studies have shown that very little medication gets absorbed into the body, so these drugs appear safe from the point of view of internal side-effects.

My five-year-old son has had eczema since he was a baby. We've managed to keep his skin reasonably comfortable with the usual moisturizers and mild steroids, but last year he had a lot of trouble with eczema around his eyes and on his cheeks. He was seen by a dermatologist who prescribed a new non-steroid eczema treatment called tacrolimus ointment. This made my son's skin feel prickly and uncomfortable shortly after it was applied for the first week he used it, but after this time he did not complain of any discomfort. The doctor had warned us that itching was a common side-effect and explained that it usually settles once the eczema improves. After a few weeks his eyelids were much better and the eczema had improved. We then only applied the ointment at night for a few weeks more and after this were able to keep things under control with a moisturizer. We still use tacrolimus ointment around his eyes and for the eczema on his face if it flares, but mostly we manage with moisturizers now.

However, there are theoretical concerns about their long-term safety, in particular whether they will increase the chances of skin cancer because of their suppressant actions on the skin's immune system. Skin cancer is already an increasingly common problem in fair skinned-people. It does not usually develop until later in life, and therefore it could take many years before a cancer-promoting effect of a new treatment becomes apparent. For this reason, pimecrolimus and tacrolimus are being used with caution at present, and are not recommended as first-line eczema treatment or for children under the age of two years.

Topical non-steroidal immunosuppressants can cause an unpleasant burning and stinging sensation shortly after being applied to eczema. This generally settles with continued use as the skin improves.

Oral and intravenous treatments

Antihistamines

Oral antihistamines are commonly used in the form of tablets and syrup as treatment for allergic reactions and itchy skin complaints. However, the itch of eczema, which is the most persistent and distressing symptom of this skin condition, is triggered by many inflammatory substances not just histamine. This probably explains why antihistamines usually have little if any effect in eczema. Although they are often prescribed, there is a lack of good scientific evidence that either the old-fashioned sedating or newer non-drowsy antihistamines are of benefit in eczema. Sedating antihistamines such as chlorpheniramine and hydroxyzine may allow eczema sufferers to get a better night's sleep because they induce drowsiness and deeper sleep, which reduce the likelihood of scratching. However, they can cause a sleepy 'hangover' the next day.

Topical antihistamines are not recommended for the treatment of eczema as they are usually ineffective and may cause allergic reactions with prolonged use. However, a topical formulation of the antihistamine-like antidepressant drug called 'doxepin' is sometimes helpful in treating very itchy, stubborn, localized patches of eczema such as lichen simplex chronicus (see Chapter 3, page 72). It is not used for widespread patterns of eczema such as atopic eczema because it gets absorbed into the body and may cause sedation and side effects on the heart.

Oral steroids

Oral corticosteroids such as prednisolone are occasionally prescribed in short courses to treat a severe eczema flare. This treatment may be justified to get someone over a flare-up at an important time such as during exams or before a wedding. Although oral steroids are usually very effective, the eczema rebounds quickly, going back to its previous severity within a week or so after they are stopped unless other treatment has been initiated to get it under control.

The dose of prednisolone is based approximately on someone's body weight, and medication should be taken first thing each day to minimize interference with production of the body's natural steroid, cortisol. Long-term use of oral steroids should be avoided because they can cause many serious side-effects such as diabetes, raised blood pressure and thinning of the bones (osteoporosis). They can also suppress growth in children. These internal problems do not apply to topical steroids, except when excessive quantities of potent or very potent steroids have been overused.

Ciclosporin

Ciclosporin is a powerful immunosuppressant drug that is taken by mouth, and is widely used to prevent rejection of transplanted organs. It has anti-inflammatory actions in the skin and has been shown to be of benefit in severe atopic eczema. However, ciclosporin treatment requires close monitoring because it can cause kidney damage and high blood pressure. This means that someone taking this drug has to have frequent blood tests and blood pressure checks. Because the risks of kidney damage increase with the length of treatment, ciclosporin is only approved in adults as a short-term treatment for up to eight weeks. It is only prescribed for severe, disabling eczema and should be used under the supervision of a specialist.

Azathioprine

Azathioprine is another immunosuppressant drug that has traditionally been used to prevent organ transplant rejection. It can be of benefit in severe eczema, and is sometimes used as a long-term treatment. Like ciclosporin, it requires very close monitoring with blood tests. Azathioprine works slowly at first, with little improvement in the first month. The main risks of azathioprine are that it can reduce the production of new blood cells in the bone marrow, leading to anaemia and a lack of infection-fighting white blood cells, which can make someone vulnerable to severe infections. Azathioprine can also cause inflammation of the liver and, occasionally, tummy upsets with nausea and vomiting. As it works by suppressing the body's immune system, there may be an increased risk of developing certain cancers, such as lymphoma, after taking it for many years. Azathioprine is only prescribed for eczema that is severe and uncontrollable with topical therapy, and should only be used under the supervision of a specialist.

Interferon gamma and high dose intravenous immunoglobulin therapy

These newer forms of eczema treatment are seldom used because they are extremely expensive and have to be given by injection or as intravenous infusions in hospital. They are part of a growing group of treatments called 'biologicals' and are concentrated forms of naturally occurring immune chemicals. They are only normally available in specialist centres, and not of any current relevance to the great majority of eczema sufferers.

Ultraviolet therapy

Many people with eczema notice that their skin improves on a sunny holiday. The main benefits of sun exposure in eczema and other inflammatory rashes are thought to come from the sun's invisible ultraviolet (UV) rays. These work by damping down the over-active immune system in the skin. Fluorescent lamps that emit UV have been used as an artificial form of sunlight therapy or 'phototherapy' for atopic eczema since the 1970s.

There are two main forms of UV phototherapy:

1. UVA – Ultraviolet radiation of relatively long wavelengths
2. UVB – Ultraviolet radiation of relatively short wavelengths.

These are administered in air-conditioned light cabinets that are like upright sunbeds and about the size of a public telephone box. Treatment is carried out in a dermatology day treatment unit and supervised directly by specialist nurses.

dermatological phototherapy
Use of light or ultraviolet rays to treat skin conditions.

Dermatological phototherapy is usually carried out two or three times a week for a four- to six-week course, and the amount of UV exposure is gradually increased over this period.

UVB treatment is used most commonly. It is given in two forms: broad band UVB and the newer narrow band UVB (also known as TLO1). UVA therapy needs to be combined with taking a plant extract called psoralen in order to be effective. This treatment is known as PUVA (Psoralen and UVA). Sunbeds in tanning parlours mainly emit UVA, but on its own this is not an effective treatment for eczema and so they are not recommended.

Dermatological phototherapy is not suitable for young children or frail elderly people who cannot stand unaided in the treatment cabinet. Repeated courses of PUVA can increase the chance of skin cancer development, especially in fair-skinned people, and consequently treatment needs to be carefully monitored. There are no proven risks of skin cancer with UVB treatment but this remains a possibility, and all phototherapy should be considered carefully, weighing up the likely risks versus the benefits for the individual.

Q Does natural sunshine help eczema?

A Exposure to natural sunshine can help eczema, although humid climates can increase sweating and aggravate the skin. When choosing a holiday, the ideal climate is sunny, warm and dry. However, not everyone benefits from the sunshine, and some people find that their eczema actually gets worse in sunny weather. There is a rare form of eczema called chronic actinic dermatitis which usually affects the face and neck area in middle-aged and elderly men, and it is caused by an allergy to sunlight.

Complementary alternative medicine

Due to the fact that most forms of eczema are chronic and incurable, some people get disillusioned with conventional medical therapy and seek answers through complementary medicine. With the exception of Chinese herbal therapy, there is little evidence that complementary therapy is of any benefit for allergic/atopic conditions, including eczema. Some studies have suggested that homeopathic immunotherapy may help in asthma, but larger analyses have not shown a consistent benefit compared with dummy treatment (placebo). This does not rule out the possibility that homeopathy can help eczema, but at the moment there is not enough evidence to support its use.

Traditional Chinese herbal medicine

Traditional Chinese herbal medicine has been practised in the Far East for many centuries. It involves using mixtures of a dozen or so dried plant parts and herbs, which are prescribed by the practitioner on an individual basis (one person's eczema treatment being different from another's). Although this sort of treatment has been found to work in atopic eczema, there are several problems:

✧ Unpleasant taste! Traditional Chinese herbal therapy is drunk as a brew made by boiling the herbs for several hours. It has an unpleasant taste that most adults find unpalatable and children are unlikely to accept.

✧ Safety concerns. Although it has been argued that Chinese herbal therapy has a longer track record than conventional medicine, there are still concerns about its safety as it has not undergone the rigorous testing that any conventional new eczema treatment has to face. Very little is known about how herbal medicines interact with other forms of medication. One particular concern is that Chinese herbal therapy has been found to cause liver abnormalities in a small number of people. Other forms of herbal treatment have been linked to kidney damage. In view of this, it is recommended that people taking Chinese herbal medication should be monitored closely with blood tests.

✧ Availability. Chinese herbal therapy is not available from conventional medical doctors or through the NHS, and it can be expensive. In the 1990s, a granule formulation of Chinese herbs was available on prescription but this product was withdrawn. One of the main problems in producing it was maintaining quality control, ensuring that exactly the same balance of herbs was used in each batch.

✧ Herbal creams and ointments are sometimes offered by people practising traditional Chinese medicine. Although they are promoted as safe, some have been found to contain potent steroids. The sale of any product containing a potent steroid is illegal in the UK where they should only be available on prescription by a registered medical practitioner.

✧ Aloe vera has been used as a herbal remedy for wounds and burns, and may help skin healing. However, there is very little evidence that it helps eczema and it is often used in gel formulations which can be drying.

Q I'd like to try herbal therapy for my child's eczema as it seems much more natural than steroid creams and drugs. My friend has recently bought a pot of herbal cream which helped clear her eczema. However, I've heard some reports that herbal treatment can be harmful so this is quite confusing.

A Plants contain many active substances, and some of these can help treat ailments and illnesses. However, it would be wrong to assume that everything that comes from a herb or plant is safe because it is natural. Some of our most dangerous poisons and drugs come from plants and are very natural! Plant extracts can cause allergic reactions and are not recommended in the treatment of eczema.

Q I'd like to try aromatherapy. Is this safe for my eczema?

A Aromatherapy involves the use of concentrated essences (essential oils) from flowers, herbs and trees to treat a range of health problems. These fragrances smell lovely and can aid relaxation and reduce stress, but there is no evidence that they are of any specific benefit in eczema. The carers of young children with eczema may get relief from the soothing effects of an aromatherapy massage, but dermatologists do not recommend that aromatherapy oils are used directly on eczema skin as they may cause irritation and allergic reactions.

CHAPTER

7

Taking control

Coping with eczema

In spite of progress in our understanding of eczema, this remains for most people a chronic (long-term) and sometimes incurable complaint. It can be difficult to adjust to life with any chronic problem, but with help eczema sufferers and their families can learn to cope effectively with this condition.

Feeling in control

One of the common causes of stress or a low mood is having a persistent problem and not feeling in control or able to cope with it. Simply putting on a brave face for the outside world is not the answer. You will feel more in control of your eczema if you are well informed about its cause, triggers, and understand the different treatment options available. If you are not sure how to use your treatment, ask your doctor or nurse specialist to spend some time explaining this. Try to work with (not against) your doctors and nurses to manage your eczema most effectively. If, like most people, you have a chronic form of eczema, do not build up false hope of a magic cure, but try to accept this as a problem you can learn to live with. Focus your energy on using your treatment regularly and think if there are any ways of changing your lifestyle that could help your skin.

Sharing your problems

Don't suffer in silence. Explain to your friends, family, work or school about how eczema may affect your daily activities, and find someone you feel comfortable with to talk about your problems. Unfortunately, eczema sufferers often complain that their doctors are unaware of just how much eczema affects them. Worse still, some feel that their doctor is just not interested. This is a great pity, because having confidence in your doctor and a good relationship with them is as much a part of treatment as the medication they prescribe. If friends and family can't help in this way, consider joining a self-help group where you can talk with other eczema sufferers.

Stress and eczema

Eczema is not directly caused by stress, although it is possible that stress makes eczema worse, and eczema can certainly be stressful. Many eczema sufferers say that their skin flares up after emotional conflict or with worry and anxiety such as around the time of exams. There is no one answer to managing stress, and we all need to find our own ways of coping with it. For one person, this may be by going out with a group of friends, whereas another person may unwind better by being alone and listening to music or reading.

Lifestyle choices

Young people with eczema need to think carefully about their choice of career as certain occupations put added strain on the skin through exposure to irritants (see Chapter 4, page 75) or low humidity. Try to lead as full and normal a life with regard to your social life and hobbies. For example, you may need to allow extra time in the changing room to apply creams after playing sport or going to the gym. Cigarette smoke can irritate eczema on exposed body sites, particularly the face, apart from having so many other harmful effects, so try and avoid smoky places. Alcohol in excess can also cause skin dehydration and lead to an eczema flare.

Key messages

✧ Stress does not cause eczema but it can make it worse.

✧ Take control of your treatment: understand how, where and when to use different creams and ointments – become your own expert.

✧ Tell your doctor or nurse how you feel and ask them to explain any treatment you do not understand.

Problems with children and teenagers

When a child has eczema the whole family's life can be affected because of disturbed sleep, special diets and the time and attention needed for treatment and visits to the doctor. However, one benefit for the parents is that these children are often bright and highly intelligent. Remember that most children's eczema improves as they grow up and that children do not usually dwell on past or future problems. Keep a positive outlook about your child's skin complaint, although this may be difficult at times, and everyone will cope better.

Atopic eczema often improves in teenagers once puberty starts and the skin becomes oilier. It may persist, however, and cause particular problems in this age group because of its impact on appearance and choice of clothing at a time in life when these are very important to the individual. Adolescents are often extremely self-conscious about any skin complaints, especially on visible sites such as the hands and face. Some young people go through a rebellious phase where they give up their treatment as an act of protest. Extra patience, understanding and support may be needed in managing eczema in this age group in order to help the individual cope with their chronic skin condition and to accept responsibility for its treatment.

my experience

I have a four-year-old son, Thomas, who has quite bad eczema, and a two-year-old, George, who has great skin. I was having problems finding the extra time and attention necessary to put all the creams and ointments on Thomas, as whenever I tried to do this George would play up, especially in the evenings when everyone's patience runs low. I was advised not to use bubble baths because these could upset Thomas's skin, but found out that it was OK for the boys to share a bath with bath oils and use emollients to wash. Thomas gets out of the bath first, which gives me some extra time to apply a steroid on any active areas of eczema before giving him his moisturizer to put on. We dab the moisturizer all over and play join the dots or draw smiley faces on his tummy. I also put a few dots of moisturizer on George so he doesn't feel left out. I try and make bathtime as much fun as possible without allowing them to flood the floor!

Thomas gets more attention in the daytime with all his treatment and special clothing, so I try to set aside some one-to-one time when I can make things up to George. It's not easy trying to get a fair balance of attention when one child has special needs, and I sometimes feel pulled in all directions. However, I appreciate that this is a difficult time and that as the children get older we will be able to talk things through together to try and avoid feelings of jealousy.

Q Which fabrics should people with eczema A wear?

The roughness of fabric next to the skin is a very important consideration for eczema sufferers because their skin is more easily irritated. In order to keep comfortable they need to choose the fabric of their clothing carefully. Although pure cotton is usually recommended, the inherent roughness or finish of a fabric seems to be more important than whether it is natural or synthetic. Fabrics should be absorbent and allow moisture to escape as sweating can aggravate eczema. New garments should be washed before use to remove any chemicals in case these cause skin irritation. However, it is not necessary to specifically use undyed, unbleached or organic cotton. Using a low fragrance conditioner can help keep clothing softer and more comfortable.

Tips for managing itching

Itching and scratching are thought to have evolved to protect the body against infestations and parasites, and they have persisted although the need has mostly passed. Many skin complaints are itchy, but few are as itchy as certain types of eczema. The itch of atopic eczema is one of the most distressing symptoms, and sufferers say they can only get relief by hard scratching or drawing blood. The itch is thought to happen because nerve fibres that usually sense pain are triggered by many of the inflammatory substances present in eczema skin. Unfortunately, there is no specific antidote to itching other than controlling the underlying eczema.

Apart from feeling unpleasant, itch in eczema is a big problem because it leads to scratching that causes further damage to the skin, making the eczema worse. This can set up a cycle of itching and scratching that can be extremely difficult to break.

Many things can trigger itch, including sudden changes in temperature, heat, sweating, low humidity, rough clothing and anxiety. Here are some simple recommendations to reduce these triggers:

✧ Keep the skin as well moisturized as possible – don't wait until it gets dry

✧ Bath water or showers should be cool to warm rather than hot

✧ Avoid overheating in bed at night – choose a light-weight duvet with soft bedclothes, and keep the bedroom well ventilated

✧ Keep fingernails cut short and filed with an emery board to remove sharp edges, and wear cotton mitts or gloves at night

✧ Wear the softest of fabrics next to your skin

and avoid anything which feels rough or is made out of wool

✧ Try to pat or pinch itchy skin rather than dig with the nails

✧ For immediate relief, gently and quickly smooth a thin layer of a cooled emollient (kept in the fridge) or a menthol-containing preparation such as 1 per cent menthol in aqueous cream

✧ Accept that children with moderate or severe atopic eczema are usually unable to control their scratching, and allow them limited periods of scratch time. Shouting or telling them off simply doesn't work.

myth

People with eczema itch when they wear wool because they are allergic to wool or lanolin.

fact

Wool itch is caused by the coarse prickly fibres present in this material and is nothing to do with an allergy. Many people with normal-looking skin are also unable to tolerate woollen garments because of irritation. There is no cure for this problem but the remedy is simply to avoid woolly or rough fabrics next to the skin.

Q What is habit reversal therapy?

A A lot of the scratching in chronic eczema is done out of habit rather than because of irritation. As families and friends often comment, someone with eczema may often be totally unaware that they are scratching. Habit reversal is a form of behavioural or psychological treatment for disorders such as tics or nail biting, and has also been shown to help chronic eczema. The first step is to make someone aware of whenever they rub, scratch or pick their skin. This identifies an individual's 'scratchy situations'. Next, the person is shown an alternative way of reacting to the scratch trigger such as counting to 30 and clenching their fists. If the urge to scratch has not gone away after this time, they are allowed to pinch their skin to get relief. Over time, this new 'desirable' behaviour takes over from the unconscious scratching behaviour, and the eczema improves once scratching diminishes. People undergoing this treatment require considerable support and follow-up. It requires time, expertise and enthusiasm, and is unfortunately not widely available.

my experience

I developed eczema in early childhood, and have now lived with it for more than 50 years. My early memories include spending weeks in hospital wrapped in bandages, and suffering with sore cracked skin on my face, arms and legs. This caused a lot of problems at school, where I was teased and called names. I felt very embarrassed about my appearance and hated changing in front of other children and playing sports. The irritation was never ending, and I would sometimes feel as if my blood was boiling and I would tear at my skin to get relief. The only thing that seemed to help the itch was scratching until I had drawn blood. I was 'lucky' in that treatment with steroid creams had recently been invented, and these provided some relief. In later life, my skin got a little better, and I learned how to use moisturizers effectively to treat the never-ending dryness. Wearing cotton next to my skin and avoiding any extremes of climate also helped. As a young man, I still felt self-conscious about my skin when meeting people at work and going out on dates. I worried that I would never get married, but thankfully met someone special who accepted my skin problems as part of me, and has been a great source of support over the years. I am now able to keep my eczema under control with simple treatment, but still need to take extra time in the bathroom every morning and evening applying creams and ointments. It took me several years to come to terms with eczema but I have now accepted that it is something I have to live with, or even that has to live with me!

CHAPTER

8

Health care for patients with eczema

The detailed infrastructure of health care systems can be a confusing subject as it varies from one country to another, and can be subject to some reorganization depending on the government in power. Politics aside, a simplified description of the health care within the UK's National Health Service (NHS) is given below that may be relevant to people with eczema.

Types of care

Primary care

This is provided within the community and is based in surgeries or health centres. The main members of the primary care team, who are involved in looking after patients with skin disease, are the general practitioners (GPs) and practice nurses. Health visitors and midwives can also advise about skin care in babies and young children.

Intermediary care

A relatively new concept in dermatology, intermediary care involves an extra tier of health care between general practice (primary care) and the hospital. It is usually based in the community and may be provided by a general practitioner with specialist interest (GPWSI). This person is a family doctor who has developed a special interest and experience in dermatology. They may work closely with a specialist dermatology nurse, and can help provide care for patients with skin problems who need some expert advice but whose conditions are not serious or severe enough to need hospital-based care.

Secondary care

This is provided in local hospitals, by teams of specialist doctors and nurses. Hospitals were traditionally divided into district general hospitals and teaching hospitals. Nowadays, teaching of undergraduate and post-graduate doctors and nurses takes place in both types of hospital and their roles are much more alike.

Medical personnel

Consultant dermatologist

The hospital dermatology team is led by a consultant dermatologist – a medically qualified doctor who has spent at least four years training specifically in dermatology. This training period must be spent in a series of recognized or accredited posts that provide a good standard of education and experience. All UK consultant dermatologists are listed on the specialist register of the General Medical Council. At present in the UK there are fewer dermatologists per capita than for most other European countries. Unfortunately this shortage of specialists is one of the factors that has led to long hospital waiting times.

Associate specialists and staff grade dermatologists

These doctors have specialized in dermatology and often have many years of experience in dermatology, but for one reason or another cannot fulfil all of the requirements for entry into the specialist register.

Clinical assistants

These are mostly general practitioners with a special interest who spend some of their time in hospital-based clinics, and usually work closely with a consultant.

Specialist registrars

Specialist registrars (SPRs) are qualified doctors who are training in a particular specialty in order to become a consultant. Their training covers all the main aspects of dermatology and involves being on call for emergency referrals from primary care and casualty.

Senior house officer

Senior house officers (SHOs) are qualified doctors who are gaining further experience in different medical or surgical specialties. They usually work under the immediate supervision of a specialist registrar.

Pre-registration house officer

A pre-registration house officer (PRHO) has qualified as a doctor and is in their first year of work as a hospital doctor.

Dermatology secretary

Hospital-based teams are supported by dedicated secretaries who help to organize the day-to-day running of the department, deal with telephone enquiries and type clinic letters. They do not usually organize or reschedule NHS appointments because other administrative staff do this.

Dermatology specialist nurses

These are qualified nurses who have special expertise in treating skin conditions. They are usually the main professionals who provide dermatology day treatment, including ultraviolet phototherapy. Some nurses also work in clinics, treating minor complaints like warts, and running education clinics to explain and monitor eczema treatments such as topical therapy and wet wraps. Nurses may also be able to prescribe certain drugs, including emollients and carry out simple operations.

Dermatology liaison nurses

These nurses work both in the hospital and in the community, and play a very helpful role in the management of young children with eczema as they can provide the family with advice and support at home.

Pharmacists

Pharmacists may be based in hospitals or the community. They dispense prescription-only drugs and 'over-the-counter' medication, and can give advice on the treatment of minor skin complaints. Many products for eczema treatment, including mild steroids, can be bought over the counter without prescription.

Prescription charges

In the UK, a set charge is levied for each item on a prescription. This is the same whatever the size or cost of the item. Some eczema treatment such as emollients, moisturizers and bath oils can be bought without prescription, but this usually works out more expensive if large quantities are required. Many people are exempt from paying prescription charges, including children, the elderly and pregnant women. Eczema treatment can be expensive for people who pay for their own prescriptions, and it is often worth paying a fixed annual charge that covers all prescribed medication for this period.

The NHS appointment system

This is an area that is under change. Traditionally, when a person was referred to hospital, their doctor would send a letter to the specialist who would then prioritize how quickly they needed to be seen. The patient would then be sent an appointment for their clinic visit. A major problem with this system was that when waiting times were very long, people often failed to turn up for their appointments because they forgot, saw another doctor, or got better and were unable to contact the clinic to cancel their appointment. In order to reduce the number of missed appointments, some hospitals have now instituted a different system where people's names are put on a waiting list and they are only told of their appointment date a few weeks beforehand. In some surgeries, the doctor is now able to arrange their patient's appointment directly with the hospital by computer.

Further help

Allergy UK
Deepdene House
30 Bellegrove road
Welling
Kent
DA14 3PY
www.allergyuk.org
Tel: 0208 3038525

American Academy of Dermatology

This website has a public resources section.
www.aad.org

Best treatments

Clinical evidence from the British Medical Journal.
www.besttreatments.co.uk

British Association of Dermatologists

This website has a public resources section.
www.bad.org.uk

Disability living allowance for sufferers or carers with atopic eczema on low income
Tel: 0800 882200

National Eczema Society
Hill House
Highgate Hill
London
N19 5NA
Email: helpline@eczema.org
www.eczema.org
Helpline: 0870 241 3604

National Health Service (NHS) Direct
www.nhsdirect.nhs.uk
Helpline: 0845 4647

Glossary

acute eczema   Eczema that has recently started or flared up (over hours or days). The skin is hot, red, swollen, itchy and sore.

allergen   A natural or manmade substance which is misidentified as harmful by some people's immune systems, leading to an allergic reaction.

allergic sensitization   When someone's immune system has identified an allergen as 'harmful' and the person is therefore at risk of getting symptoms of an allergic reaction when they are exposed to the allergen.

antibodies   Natural substances produced by white blood cells which help to fight infection.

atopic eczema   An endogenous or constitutional type of eczema that usually starts in babies or children who have a family tendency to eczema, asthma and hay fever. It is extremely itchy and is normally worse in the skin folds.

bacterial colonization   When low levels of bacteria are present on the skin without causing any disease.

candida   A family of yeast that can infect warm, moist skin areas, such as the skin folds around the groin, to cause soreness and redness (thrush).

chronic disease	A long lasting health problem, which may be incurable. This term relates to the duration of the disease, not to how severe it is.
chronic eczema	Eczema that has been present for a long time (weeks or months), and is repeatedly scratched. The skin looks thickened, lined and flaky, and is feels dry, itchy and sore.
cradle cap	A common minor skin complaint in newborn and young babies caused by a build-up of scaly skin in the scalp.
creams	Preparations containing a mixture of oil and water that are used to treat skin complaints and may act as moisturizers. They usually look white.
cytokines	Natural messenger substances produced by many different cells in the body, including white blood cells and skin cells. They help to activate defence mechanisms against infection and aid healing.
delayed food allergy	This happens about 6–24 hours after eating the food, and can cause an eczema flare, scratching, tummy pain and diarrhoea. There is no simple test to confirm this diagnosis, but a food diary may help, and suspect foods can be excluded under the supervision of a dietician.
delayed type allergy	An allergy reaction that starts hours or days after exposure to the allergen.
dermatological phototherapy	Use of light or ultraviolet rays to treat skin conditions.
dermis	The deeper layer of the skin that contains blood and tissue fluid to nourish and heal the skin, and a network of tough and stretchy fibres to give the skin strength.
disease signs	The outward appearance of a disease which can be observed by someone else, for example a rash, or more specific features such as redness, swelling, blisters, scaling.
disease symptoms	The uncomfortable sensations that a person feels, for example pain and itching.
emollients and moisturizers	Soothing preparations that help the skin retain moisture and improve dryness.

epidermis	The outer layer of the skin which is constantly being renewed and is made up of layer upon layer of skin cells (keratinocytes). These grow outwards to the surface where they die and are shed.
eczema/dermatitis	An inflammatory rash which is red, swollen and blistered, or scaly and itchy.
eczema flare	When eczema becomes active, looking red and swollen or dry, and feeling hot and itchy.
endogenous (constitutional) eczema	Eczema that occurs due to an inbuilt tendency and not primarily because of something in the outside world.
erythema	Skin redness due to increased blood flow in the dermis.
exogenous (contact) eczema	Eczema that is caused by skin contact with an external substance.
herpes simplex	This is the virus that causes cold sores. It can lead to a widespread painful infection in children or adults with atopic eczema called 'eczema herpeticum'.
hives or urticaria	This is an itchy, bumpy, swollen rash that looks like a nettle rash.
immediate food allergy	This happens within minutes to an hour or two, and causes swollen lips, hives, scratching, sneezing, wheezing, vomiting or collapse. The diagnosis can be confirmed by allergy tests. Allergy-provoking foods must be strictly avoided.
immune system	The body's defence system which is made up of many specialized cells that circulate through the skin, blood and glands, and have evolved to recognize and fight disease and infection.
immunoglobulin E/ IgE	A type of infection-fighting antibody made by white blood cells which is overproduced in people with atopic conditions. It can trigger allergic reactions when the body comes into contact with an allergen.
immuno-suppressant	An agent that reduces the activity of the body's immune system.
infected eczema	Eczema which has an added infection, usually with the bacteria *Staph aureus*. Infected eczema looks red, 'angry' and weepy with yellow crusts or spots, and feels itchy and sore.

inflammation	A process where more blood cells and infection-fighting substances are present in part of the body. In the skin this causes redness, heat, swelling and soreness or irritation. All these features are present in eczema.
irritant	A harsh external substance or climate that damages the skin.
keratinocytes	The skin cells that make up most of the epidermis. They contain a tough protein called 'keratin'.
leg ulcers	These are non-healing wounds on the lower legs which may be caused by circulatory problems. Venous leg ulcers occur because of raised pressure and sluggish blood flow in the veins.
moisturizers and emollients	Soothing preparations that help the skin retain moisture and improve dryness.
mycology tests	Analysis for fungal infections, usually done on scrapings of the skin or nail clippings.
occlusive dressings	These cover the skin closely and trap moisture. They can help treatment work more effectively on dry, thickened areas of skin.
ointments	Greasy preparations that keep moisture in the skin and improve dry skin complaints.
patch tests	Skin allergy tests to investigate possible allergic contact eczema.
pityrosporum	A yeast which normally lives on oily areas of skin. If the natural balance of microbes on the skin is upset, the yeast can overgrow and trigger seborrhoeic eczema.
prevalence	The proportion of people with a condition in a defined population.
pruritus	An unpleasant itchy or prickling sensation that makes you want to scratch.
psoriasis	A skin complaint that causes red patches with thick silvery scales and cracks. It usually affects the skin over joints and the scalp, and often runs in families.
sebum	Skin grease which is made by sebaceous glands in the skin. These glands become active at puberty and are abundant on the face, scalp and upper torso.

skin irritant	A harsh substance that can damage the skin. Irritants are classified as strong or weak irritants depending on how harmful they are.
skin lipids	Natural oily substances produced by the skin to help moisturize the outer layer and prevent drying.
skin prick tests	Tests carried out on the skin to demonstrate immediate type allergies.
Staphylococcus aureus	A bacteria which overgrows on the skin of people with atopic eczema and can lead to eczema flares and skin infections.
steroid atrophy	Thinning of the skin due to the use of a topical steroid or from taking high doses of steroids internally.
stratum corneum	The outermost layer of the epidermis which is made of flat, dead skin cells (keratinocytes). It acts as the skin's main protective barrier, keeping moisture locked in and harmful substances out.
tinea	A ringworm type fungus that can infect the outer layers of the skin, nails and hair.
topical treatment	A treatment that is applied to the surface of the body rather than being taken internally.
urticaria or hives	This is an itchy, bumpy, swollen rash that looks like a nettle rash.
venous eczema	Eczema on the lower legs around the ankles which is due to underlying varicose or blocked veins.
venous hypertension	Raised pressure of blood in the veins of the lower legs.

Index

acute eczema 14
adult eczema
  asteototic (dry) eczema 13,
    71–2
  atopic eczema 21, 24, 58–62,
    77
  discoid eczema 13, 14, 65–6,
    110
  endogenous hand and foot
    eczema 67–9
  lichen simplex 72–3, 106,
    113
  seborrhoeic eczema 13, 14,
    62–5
  venous eczema 69–71, 86
adult eczema ix, 58–73
alcohol 122
allergens 12
  and allergic contact eczema 54,
    55, 81, 83
  and atopic eczema 26–8, 29,
    59, 60
  house dust mites 33–5
  and patch tests 92, 94
  sunlight 116
  and topical steroids 109

allergic contact eczema (ACE) 12,
    13, 74, 75, 81–6
  causes of 82–3
  in children 54–6, 83
  testing for 87–8
  treatment 83–6
allergic desensitization 36–7
allergic sensitization 28
allergy tests 15–16, 87–96
  cosmetic allergies 94–5
  delayed allergy reactions 87–8,
    91–6
  immediate allergy reactions
    88–91
  see also blood tests; patch
    testing; skin prick tests
aloe vera 118
anaphylactic shock 44
animal fur allergies 27, 35–6
  testing for 88, 90
antibiotics 32, 98, 110–11
  and leg ulcers 71
  and nappy rash 20
  resistance to 50
  and Staph aureus infection
    49–50

antibodies 9
antihistamines 28, 112–13
  and patch tests 93
antiperspirants 78
antiseptics 49, 50, 71, 103
aromatherapy 119
asathioprine 114–15
asteototic (dry) eczema 14, 71–2
asthma 23, 25, 88, 90
athlete's foot 66
atopic eczema 13, 14
  in adults 21, 24, 58–62
    atopic facial eczema 59,
      61–2
    atopic hand eczema 59,
      60–1
    and irritant contact eczema
      77
    signs and symptoms of 58–9
    triggers for 59
  and allergens 26–8
  and antibiotics 110, 113
  in children
    allergy tests for 88
    causes of 28–30
    and diet 37–46
    frequency of 24
    growing out of 24, 26
    and the home environment
      30–7
    and infection 46–53
    outcomes 25–6
    and quality of life 25–6
    and soap 101
  in children x, 21–38
  managing the itch 124–6

babies 18–21, 83
  atopic eczema 21
  breastfeeding 19, 31, 38–9
  cradle cap 18–19, 20
  and formula milk 39–40
  nappy rash 19–21, 77
  weaning and infant feeding 40
bacteria 2, 47
  and ointments 101
  probiotic 32
  and skin swabs 47–8

bandages 103–4
bath oils 102
beds and bedding 34
blisters, pompholyx hand and foot
      eczema 67–8
blood flow 6–7
blood tests 17, 28, 45, 87, 90–1
breastfeeding 19, 31, 38–9
bubble bath 102

cancer 112, 115, 116
candida (thrush) 20
childhood eczema
  allergic contact eczema 54–6,
      83
  atopic eczema x, 21–38, 101
  coping with 16, 122
  diagnosis 15–16
  lip lick eczema 56
  newborn and young babies
      18–21
  and stinging ointments/creams
      85
  and topical steroids 56, 57, 106
childhood eczema ix, 18–57, 127
Chinese herbal medicine 117–18
chronic eczema 14, 121
ciclosporin 114
clothing 123, 124
cold sores 51–2
collagen 7
complementary medicine 117–19
conjunctivitis 88
contact eczema 12, 74–85
  see also allergic contact eczema;
      irritant contact eczema
costs of eczema ix
cradle cap 18–19, 20
creams 102
cytokines 9

dandruff 63
dark skins 14, 15
delayed allergy reactions
  food allergies 44–5
  testing for 87–8, 91–6
deodorants 78
dermatitis 9

dermatology nurses 104
dermis (deeper skin) 6–8
diet
  and childhood atopic eczema
    37–46
  see also food allergies
discoid eczema 13, 14, 65–6,
    110
disease signs and symptoms 14
doctors 121, 127, 128–9
doxepin 113
dust mites *see* house dust mite
    allergies

earrings 83
eczema
  diagnosis 15–16
  different types of 11–14
  signs and symptoms 14–15
  what it is 9–11
eczema flare 27, 44
  steroid treatment for 113–14
eczema herpeticum 51–2
emollients 97, 98–104, 126
  added ingredients 103
  and allergic contact eczema 83,
    84
  application 100
  choosing 100–1
  and irritant contact eczema 79,
    80
  and topical steroids 107
  see also moisturizers
endogenous (constitutional)
    eczema 12, 13–14, 15,
    67–9
epidermis (outer layer of skin)
    3–6, 9–10
erythema 10
essential fatty acids 30
exclusion diets 41–2, 91
exogenous eczema *see* contact
    eczema
eyelids
  and atopic facial eczema 61–2
  and irritant contact eczema
    77–8
  and skin thinning 7

face eczema 16
  atopic facial eczema 59, 61–2
fingertip eczema 69
fingertip unit 108
flooring 34, 36
food additives 43
food allergies
  and adult eczema 59
  and breastfeeding 39
  and childhood atopic eczema
    23–4, 42–6
  delayed 44–5
  exclusion diets 41–2, 91
  and formula milk 39–40
  immediate 43–4, 45
  and infant feeding 41
  intolerance 42–3
  testing for 88, 90–1
foot eczema 14, 110
  athlete's foot 66
  endogenous hand and foot
    eczema 67–9
  juvenile plantar dermatitis 57
formula milk 39–40, 41
fragrance allergies 95–6

genes 13, 29
glucocorticosteroids 104
goat milk 40
growth in children, and atopic
    eczema 46

habit reversal therapy 125
hair dye allergies 85
hand eczema 14, 16, 110
  adult atopic 59, 60–1
  endogenous hand and foot
    eczema 67–9
  irritant 76
hay fever 23, 25, 26–7, 81, 90
health care systems 127–31
herbal medicine 117–19
herpes simplex 46, 51–2
histamines 28, 93
HIV (Human Immunodeficiency
    Virus) 64
hives (nettle rash) 44, 87, 88
hospital treatment 128–30

house dust mite allergies 33–5,
        62
    testing for 88, 90
humectants 103
hygiene hypothesis 30–2
hyperkeratotic (thick skin) hand and
        foot eczema 68–9

immediate allergy reactions
    food allergies 43–4, 45
    testing for 88–91
immune system 12
    and atopic eczema 29
    and the hygiene hypothesis
        31–3
    and *Staph aureus* infection
        48
    and topical calcineurin inhibitors
        (TCIs) 111–12
    and warts 53
immunosuppressant agents 111,
        114–15
impetigo 46
imunoglobulin E 27
infantile seborrhoeic dermatitis 19,
        20
infection
    and antibiotics 110–11
    and atopic eczema 46–53
    eczema as non-infectious 10
inflammation 7, 9
interferon gamma 115
intermediary care 128
intravenous immunoglobin therapy
        115
irritant contact eczema 12, 13, 74,
        75–80
    causes of 75–6
    nappy rash 19–21, 77
    occupational risk 76
    signs and symptoms of 78
    treatment 79–80
    work-related 80
itching
    tips for managing 124–6
    and topical steroids 105

juvenile plantar dermatitis 56

keratinocytes 3, 5, 9, 10

lactose intolerance 42
Langerhans cells 6
lanolin allergy 86
latex allergy 60, 61
    testing for 89, 90
leg ulcers 71, 86
lichen simplex 72–3, 106, 113
lifestyle choices 122
lip lick eczema 56
lotions 102–3

mast cells 27–8, 88
medical personnel 128–30
melanin 5
metal allergy 54, 55, 83
milk
    breast milk 19, 31, 38–9
    cow's milk protein 39–40, 41,
        45
    formula 39–40, 41
moisturizers 97, 98–104
    application 100
    and asteototic eczema 72
    choosing 100–1
    creams 102
    and fingertip eczema 68–9
    and hand and foot eczema 68
    and irritant contact eczema 77,
        80
    lanolin allergies 86
    and lichen simplex 73
    lotions 102–3
    ointments 101–2
    and topical steroids 110
    and venous eczema 70
    see also emollients
Molluscum contagiosum 52–3
MRSA infection 50

nappy rash 19–21, 77
nelanocytes 5
nettle rash 44, 87, 88
NHS (National Health Service)
    appointment system 131
    medical personnel 128–30
    prescriptions 100, 131

non-steroidal immunosuppressants
111–2
nurses 104, 128, 130
nutritional deficiencies 45

occlusive dressings 68
occupational risk 60, 122
  of contact eczema 76, 79–80
  ointments 85, 101–2
  oral steroids 49–50, 113–14

patch testing 55–6, 67, 83, 84,
  91–4, 109
pet allergies *see* animal fur allergies
pharmacists 109, 130
pierced ears 83
pinecrolimus 111–2
pityriasis alba 15
pityrosporum yeast 64–5
pompholyx (blistering) hand and
  foot eczema 67–8
prednisolone 113–14
pregnancy 31, 38
primary care 127
probiotics 32
proteases 10
pruritus 10
psoriasis 63, 66

rhinitis 33, 88
rice milk 40
ringworm 8, 65–6

scabies 11
scratching 10, 29, 48, 105
  and lichen simplex 72–3
  and *Staph aureus* infection 48
sebaceous glands 6
seborrhoeic eczema 13, 14, 62–5
sebum 62
secondary care 128
self-help groups 121
sharing your problems 121
skin 1–17
  dermis 6–8
  epidermis 3–6, 9
  lipids 5
  pH of 6

skin—*cont.*
  subcutis 8–9
  surface area 8
  vital functions of 2
skin cancer 112, 116
skin prick tests 28, 45, 87, 89–90
skin swabs 47–8, 51–2
skincare product allergies 84–5
sleep, disturbed 46, 59
smoking 31, 38, 122
soap 101
soft furnishings 34
soft toys 35
soya milk 40
Staphylococcus aureus 46–51
statis (venous) eczema 69–71, 86
steroids 104
steroid tablets 113–14
  see also topical steroids
stinging ointments/creams 85
stratum corneum 3–5
streptococcus 48
stress and eczema 120, 121
subcutis (deepest layer of skin)
  8–9
sun exposure 7, 115, 116
  and patch tests 93
sweat, and the skin 6
swimming 25

tacrolimus 111–2
teenagers 122–3
temperatures
  indoor 34–5
  internal body 2, 6
thrush (candida) 20
tinea (ringworm) 8, 65–6
topical calcineurin inhibitors (TCIs)
  111–12 *see also*
    non-steroidal
    immunosuppressants
topical steroids 97, 104–10, 126
  and allergic contact eczema 83,
    84
  antibiotics 32, 98, 110–11
  buying from pharmacies 109
  and childhood eczema 56, 57,
    106

topical steroids—*cont.*
  combined with antibiotics
      110–11
  and discoid eczema 65, 66
  and the eyelids 62
  and hand and foot eczema 68
  how much to use 108
  and irritant contact eczema 77,
      79
  and leg ulcers 71
  and lichen simplex 73
  and lip lick eczema 56
  and moisturizers 110
  reasons for failure of 109
  side effects of 105
  and skin thinning 7, 105, 106
  and *Staph aureus* infection 49
  strengths 106–7
  and venous eczema 70, 86
treatment 97–120
  complementary medicine
      117–19
  oral and intravenous 112–15

  topical 97–110
  ultraviolet therapy 115–16

ultraviolet therapy (UV) 93,
      115–16
urticaria (nettle rash) 44, 87, 88

varicose leg ulcers 71, 86
varicose vein eczema 13, 14, 86
venous (statis) eczema 69–71,
      86
verrucas 52
viral warts 52–3

warts 52–3
washing powders 35
water
  drinking 3
  hardness 37
wet wraps 103–4
wheat intolerance 42
wintertime (asteotic) eczema 13,
      71–2

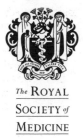

The Royal Society of Medicine (RSM) is an independent medical charity with a primary aim to provide continuing professional development for qualified medical and health-related professionals. The public benefits from health care professionals who have received high quality and relevant education from the RSM.

The Society celebrated its bicentenary in 2005. Each year it arranges and holds over 400 meetings for health care professionals across a wide range of medical subjects. In order to aid education and training further the Society also has the largest postgraduate medical library in Europe – based in central London together with online access to specialist databases. RSM Press, the Society's publishing arm, publishes books and journals principally aimed at the medical profession.

A number of conferences and events are held each year for the public as well as members of the Society. These include the successful 'Medicine and me' series, designed to bring together patients, their carers and the medical profession. In addition the RSM's Open and History of Medicine Sections arrange meetings on a regular basis which can be attended by the public.

In addition to the lectures and training provided by the RSM, members of the Society also have access to club facilities including accommodation and a restaurant. The conference and meeting facilities of the RSM were refurbished for their bicentenary and are available to the public for hire for meetings and seminars. In addition, Chandos House, a beautifully restored Georgian townhouse, designed by Robert Adam, is also now available to hire for training, receptions and weddings (as it has a civil wedding licence).

To find out more about the Royal Society of Medicine and the work it undertakes please visit www.rsm.ac.uk or call 020 7290 2991. For more information about RSM Press, please visit www.rsmpress.co.uk.